P9-DVB-531

Praise for *Awake at the Bedside*

"Marvelous. A compilation of essential treasures exploring the face and feeling of utter engagement, compassion, and wisdom in turning toward death."
—Jon Kabat-Zinn, author of *Wherever You Go, There You Are*

"Weaving together the wisdom of ancient traditions and the experience of those in the caring professions today, *Awake at the Bedside* is a deeply moving, poetic, and practical guide to dying."
—Stephen Batchelor, author of *After Buddhism*

"Profoundly moving, inspiring, and helpful, *Awake at the Bedside* is a real treasure."
—Jack Kornfield, author of *A Path with Heart*

"This is the best book I've read on the end of life—not only what it means for a dying person but what it means for all of us. Reading it moved me to tears many times."
—David Loy, author of *A New Buddhist Path*

"Important and inspirational for all us as we move into the inevitability, the necessity, the privilege, of holding space for those we love as they make their journey. It provides compassionate guidance to honor death with the same grace we do life."
—Seane Corn, yoga teacher, activist, and cofounder of Off the Mat, Into the World

"A new paradigm is expressed here: death is as important a transition as birth, the journey that needs above all else love, presence, and listening. This book speaks eloquently to this new expansion of human compassion."
—Dorothy Dai En Friedman, Zen teacher at Ocean Zendo

"From poetry, meditation, and philosophical counsel to care-giving and care-receiving guidance, this profoundly moral book is a gift to all. Vital reading for anyone involved in the process of death—and that means everybody."
—Janet Gyatso, PhD, Hershey Professor of Buddhist Studies, Harvard Divinity School

"This book isn't about sickness or death—it's about diving into the heart of life discovered when we truly meet another person. Providing practical support, emotional resonance, and celebration of ordinary sacredness, it is a priceless treasure."
—Acharya Judith Simmer-Brown, PhD, Distinguished Professor of Contemplative and Religious Studies, Naropa University

"Supportive and honest, this collection of stories, poems, and practices is a perfect companion for providing loving support to those we care for—including ourselves."
—Michael Stone, guiding teacher at True North Insight

"In the practice of medicine in the US, the act of dying has been completely separated from the care of the patient, yet this process can give one the deepest of gifts—an insight into what living a life really means. This wonderful volume will not only relieve our anxiety and fear but will allow us to embrace what is at the end of the path; it will allow our own awakening."
—James R. Doty, MD, founder and director of the Center for Compassion and Altruism Research and Education

"We experience advanced illness with such a complex and changing interplay of suffering and solace, stress and resilience, that the most certain observation is that each is unique, and one never knows what is needed, unless there is engagement. *Awake at the Bedside* illustrates that the necessary and very human task of connecting with another is one of the most important things to be learned from the practices of contemplative care."
—Dr. Russell K. Portenoy, chief medical officer, MJHS Hospice and Palliative Care

"*Awake at the Bedside* is an essential book that points out the therapeutic power of being fully present and compassionate at the beside of those who are dying."
—Dr. Mitchell Levy, medical director of the Medical Intensive Care Unit at Rhode Island Hospital

"Finally a compendium that gets us above, below, and behind the clinical science that narrows and dominates our understanding of death, dying, and wellness. How do we make meaning? How do we relate self and other on this shared ride? Let's look inside these pages and see."
—Dr. BJ Miller, Zen Hospice Project

"In *Awake at the Bedside*, we are moved from suffering to peace, darkness to light, brokenness to wholeness. It is a quiet feast of small portions: poetry, wisdom, social context, and spiritual guidance. Bring it with you."
—Thomas R. Cole, PhD, University of Texas Health Science Center at Houston

"Filled with quiet insight based on years of experience, *Awake at the Bedside* extends an intimate, wise, and loving hand on behalf of those whose lives are presently coming to an end, as well as those who care for them. As our families and communities continue to age and die, this book will serve us well."
—Eihei Peter Levitt, founder and guiding teacher of the Salt Spring Zen Circle

"Here are healing guides to being present with the dying, with the survivors, and with yourself facing death wholeheartedly. Many moving and gritty stories of passing combine with meditation instructions, subtle reflections, and poetry. These illuminating encounters with death provide deep intimacy into the heart of compassion and of a caring life. This is a truly lovely and loving book."
—Taigen Dan Leighton, author of *Zen Questions*

"When Shakyamuni Buddha directed his mind to teach the Dharma and stood up from his seat under the bodhi tree, he said, 'The gate of deathlessness is open.' Then he began to walk the path of birth, living, aging, sickness, and dying for the rest of his life with all living beings. Bodhisattvas are still walking the same path today. *Awake at the Bedside* shows how bodhisattvas are working in the modern times."
—Shohaku Okumura Roshi, author of *Living by Vow*

AWAKE
AT THE
BEDSIDE

CONTEMPLATIVE TEACHINGS ON
PALLIATIVE AND END-OF-LIFE CARE

Edited and Introduced by

Koshin Paley Ellison

and

Matt Weingast

New York Zen Center for Contemplative Care

Foreword by His Holiness the Karmapa

Wisdom Publications
199 Elm Street
Somerville, MA 02144 USA
wisdompubs.org

Library of Congress Cataloging-in-Publication Data
Names: Paley Ellison, Koshin, editor.
Title: Awake at the bedside : contemplative palliative and end-of-life care / edited and introduced by Koshin Paley Ellison and Matt Weingast, New York Zen Center for Contemplative Care.
Description: Somerville : Wisdom Publications, 2016. | Includes bibliographical references and index.
Identifiers: LCCN 2015028871 | ISBN 1614291195 (pbk. : alk. paper)
Subjects: LCSH: Caring—Religious aspects—Buddhism. | Palliative treatment.
Classification: LCC BQ4570.C27 A93 2016 | DDC 294.3/4442—dc23
LC record available at http://lccn.loc.gov/2015028871

ISBN 978-1-61429-119-0 ebook ISBN 978-1-61429-142-8

20 19 18 17 16 5 4 3 2 1

Cover and interior photographs by Joshua Bright. Cover design by Phil Pascuzzo. Interior design by Gopa&Ted2. Set in Granjon LT Std 11.25/15.

Wisdom Publications' books are printed on acid-free paper and meet the guidelines for permanence and durability of the Production Guidelines for Book Longevity of the Council on Library Resources.

This book was produced with environmental mindfulness. For more information, please visit wisdompubs.org/wisdom-environment.

Printed in the United States of America.

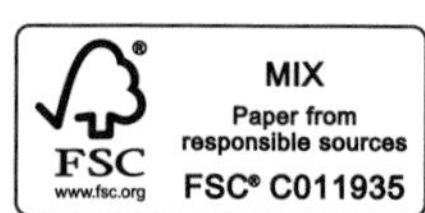

Please visit fscus.org.

For Grandma Mimi Ellison who inspired us
to bring meditation and care together as a practice,
the New York Zen Center for Contemplative Care Sangha,
Barre Center for Buddhist Studies,
our patients, their loved ones, and the clinicians
who taught us how to be with all of them

Table of Contents

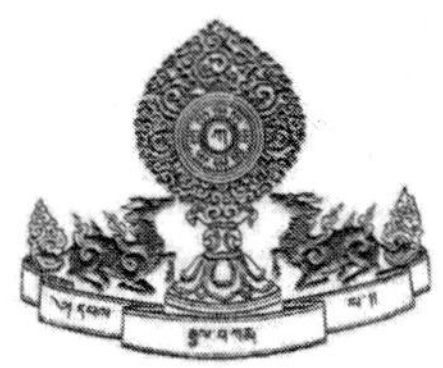

Foreword

These days many people seem to shy away from discussing death or feel great discomfort in the presence of those who are dying. Yet we need to understand that death is a natural part of life, whether it be someone else's death or our own. The diverse material in this book, accounts and reflections written from first-hand experience, will help us reflect more deeply on our attitudes to death and dying and will be of value to many people, irrespective of their religious or philosophical tradition. It shows us how, in our interactions with those who are terminally ill, we ourselves have a unique opportunity to break down the barriers of our egocentricity and fully develop our potential for an immediate, active compassion and immeasurable loving-kindness. But, of equal importance, these accounts reveal how much the dying themselves can teach us.

17th Karmapa Ogyen Trinley Dorje
Bodhgaya, India

Preface

In 1997 at the King's Highway Diner in Brooklyn, my eighty-three-year-old Grandma Mimi held up her spoon of white bean soup and said, "This is delicious. I never want to leave." Her daughter, my aunt Carol, wanted her to move to Atlanta into an assisted living home. Her son, my dad, wanted her to move to Syracuse. Mimi was still working full-time at a law office in Manhattan.

After lunch we walked back down Ocean Parkway, stopping every five minutes or so to rest on the benches. Back at her apartment, we lay on her couches, eating the caramels she adored. Suddenly she looked at me and asked, "Can I stay here with you?" I squeezed her hand and quietly said, "Yes."

So began our journey. At first there were occasional visits to doctors, then late-night ambulance rides to the hospital, and finally moving with her into hospice for the last six weeks of her life. "Do you know what's strange?" Mimi asked me late one night. "So few people who work here, or visit, seem to reflect on their lives. They're all scurrying about. Why don't they look at me? Why is there so much fear in being with another person?"

Among the caregivers around my grandma were my fellow Zen practitioners, including my future husband and coteacher Robert Chodo Campbell. Once people met her, they felt loved by her and kept showing up to sit, sing, and give her the manicures and pedicures she loved. One evening, four weeks into our stay at the hospice, she said, "Call the family and your friends. I think tonight is the night I'm going to die." After four hours of quiet sitting, she peeked at her watch, sat up, and said, "It isn't going to happen. Let's order out for pizza—you all must be hungry."

I stayed with her for the entire six weeks that she was in hospice, sleeping in a chair at the side of her bed and sometimes climbing in next to her when she seemed frightened or confused. One night she woke me and said, "I'm so sorry. I spent so many years thinking I knew what love was, but I didn't know anything. I was afraid of what I didn't understand about you. To love someone is to love everything about them, even the parts I don't understand or feel comfortable with. Part of me contracted from loving you because of your Zen practice. I felt it was a betrayal of our Jewish heritage. Please forgive me."

"For what?" I asked her.

"For not loving you completely," she said. "The way I do now. I now see that there is something so direct about your Zen practice that allows you to be with me in this way. You and Chodo should start an organization that helps people learn about meditation and how to care for people. Learning how to reflect on life and how we are spending our time is the most important thing. Please teach people. Please care for them."

On the morning of June 23, we awoke together to see the light on the tree outside the window. "Beautiful morning," she said. "Go get the *New York Times* and a coffee, sit out in the park, and enjoy the morning." She looked at me, I looked at her. We embraced, squeezed each other's hands, and I kissed her cheek. I wept. I didn't want to leave. I kissed her again on her forehead and walked out.

I sat in the park opposite the hospital in the morning sunshine, drinking my coffee and trying to read the Sunday *Times*. My cell phone rang. It was our favorite hospice nurse. "Baby, Mimi just died. Take your time and then come over."

I leaned back on the bench and craned my head to the sky. The branches in the trees were swaying in the morning breeze. A young girl was bouncing a rainbow-colored ball. An elderly man was on the next bench basking in the sun. I felt like my chest was going to burst open.

I called Chodo from her bedside. It was almost impossible to get the words out. "She's gone," I said. "Please come here right now." I squeezed Mimi's hands. They were no longer warm, and on the windowsill the stargazer lilies she loved so much had opened fully.

We washed her body, chanted, and stayed to witness the funeral director shrouding her and whisking her down the hall. I thought of the Zen teaching that talks about how all we need to do is allow ourselves and the world to change. Easy to say, I thought. And yet, here I was in the midst of my experience of fullness of the pain, grief, love, and joy of my grandma's death. Everything did change.

Everything I teach now I learned from my relationship with Mimi. Being deeply in relationship changes the world. I didn't know then that my life would pivot to teaching others and to being with many, many Mimis.

Chodo and I changed our lives and began our vision for the New York Zen Center for Contemplative Care, a nonprofit organization that offers direct care and trains people to turn toward life's great challenges: old age, illness, and dying. Everything we do is grounded in the meditation practice that helped to nourish my Hungarian Jewish grandma. This book you are holding is an expression of Grandma Mimi's blessing and love—all proceeds will go back to support the center she urged us to create. May the integration of contemplative practice and caregiving serve and heal you and all those you care for.

Koshin Paley Ellison

Introduction

This book isn't about dying. It's about life and what life has to teach us. It's about caring and what giving care really means.

The potential for intimacy—for truly being in relationship—is always available, but it can reach another level toward the end of life. Who exactly is giving care and who exactly is receiving care has the opportunity to all somehow get lost in the mix. When time is running out, caring is the only thing that matters or makes sense between beings now in the world, soon out—this giving and receiving, this intimate sharing of our inherent fragility and limited time.

A good friend of ours likes to say about her early days in caregiving that she, like much of the world, was "full of good intentions and imperfect knowledge." She had no idea what to say or what not to say, what to do or what not to do, when to ask for help, how to communicate with medical staff, patients, or family. She knew that just being there was the most important thing, but she felt utterly uncertain around anything other than quietly sitting in a chair near the head of the bed.

Perhaps you have long supported, or are just now considering supporting, those heading off to, as Shakespeare put it, that "undiscover'd country from whose bourn no traveler returns." Or maybe you're dying. Or maybe you're a relative, friend, or loved one of someone who is dying. This book, hopefully, will help. Help to comfort, help to support, help to instruct, help to inspire, and hopefully just help you to feel less alone.

The bedside can sometimes be a really lonely place—even though you're never actually alone there. To that end, we've included pieces that are appropriate for reading to the person whose bed you're alongside of.

Here you'll find pieces by some of the pioneers of palliative, contemplative, and end-of-life care, as well as many contemporary voices: doctors, Dharma teachers, chaplains, poets, and caregivers of all kinds offering specific instructions and personal accounts of some very high-level being and doing at the bedside. There are pieces here to wake you up in the morning and pieces to tuck you in when it's time for bed, pieces to hold your hand through long sleepless nights and pieces to watch with you when you don't know what you're watching for. There are poems to cry with you when you're sad, and poems to lift you up when you need lifting up. This is a book to keep you company as you make your way to the bedside, and this is a book to comfort and console as you make your way back home.

Put simply, this book is a companion. It hopes to model and encourage and support the deep intimacy that can arise through a mutual willingness to care and be cared for—evidence not only that waking up is possible, but that it is actually happening. The giving and receiving of care that is both a means toward and an expression of waking up.

In the end, when there's nothing left to hold on to—when everything else is being let go of—kindness, compassion, and love are really all that remain. These are the qualities that awaken at the bedside.

May this book help to awaken awe, respect, acceptance, and love for yourself and for all those around you—the living, the dying, and everyone anywhere in between. And may this book be of use and of comfort. The work you do, rest absolutely assured, you do for all of us.

Kozan Ichikyo

Empty-handed I entered
the world,
Barefoot I leave it.
My coming, my going—
Two simple happenings
That got entangled.

1 Transforming the Care of Serious Illness

Diane Meier

Although the world is full of suffering, it is also full of the overcoming of it.
—Helen Keller

Where do we want—where do we really want—the healthcare of death and dying to be? And how do we get there? To answer that question, we first need to look at how we arrived where we are today.

In a very short period of time, what for all of human history had been the central, shared, social experience—the inevitability and universality of death—disappeared from public view in the blink of an evolutionary eye. Here's why: Around thirty thousand years ago, life expectancy was thirty. You could die in a storm. You could die of an infection. You could die because somebody killed you. Life was a dangerous thing.

It wasn't until the development of agriculture, about ten thousand years ago, that things started to change. Soon after, people recognized that they got sick less often if they separated drinking water from sewage. In a relatively short time, the human race experienced a twenty-to-thirty-year gain in life expectancy.

Right now in this country the median age of death is seventy-eight years. So we've seen very rapid, dramatic, almost incomprehensible evolutionary change in the last one hundred years.

All of a sudden, there's no longer an expectation that death is normal or routine. In fact, death is the exception. Death itself should be defeated. Everyone thinks they deserve a long life, and that it's normal to have a long life. This idea has essentially created a market for medical care, and we've seen exponential growth in hospitals, procedures, medicines, technology, health insurance to pay for all of it, and market forces that have both caused and been the result of this huge growth in an industry. If you look at the National Institutes of Health, which has billions of dollars of taxpayer money, you could be forgiven for thinking that its mission is to eliminate death at all costs—as if somehow that is a rational social goal. I'm not writing this to be funny. This is the society in which we live.

Some people, of course, saw this as maybe not an unalloyed good. Interestingly most of them were women—middle-aged women.

After World War II, Cicely Saunders was initially a social worker and then a nurse. When a pain expert in London told her that if she wanted to have any real power and authority she had to go to medical school, she did. So she was a social worker, nurse, physician, and also a very spiritual person—an interdisciplinary team in one person. In 1967 she established St. Christopher's Hospice—the first modern hospice—almost entirely with charitable money.

She was also friends with Florence Wald, the dean of the Yale School of Nursing at the time. Cicely gave lectures at Yale, and Florence spent a sabbatical at St. Christopher's in study and practice. Then Florence went back home and established the first hospice in the United States: the Connecticut Hospice.

Elisabeth Kübler-Ross was a psychiatrist at the University of Chicago who did a very revolutionary thing. Do you know what she's remembered for? The least important thing she did: the five stages of grief. But the reason her book is so powerful is that all it is, is her listening to patients and families and quoting them. Asking them about their experience. You can't find another book that is devoted entirely to the voices of patients like that one is. *That's* what she should be remembered for; it was so revolutionary. Before this, the patient had all but disappeared. The patient was the object or the means for this marketplace to go on but was no longer at the center, and she put the patient back at the center. We owe her a huge debt of gratitude for that.

In one of my favorite quotes from Cicely Saunders—a masterpiece of understatement—she said, "Many of the patients feel deserted by their doctors at the end. Ideally the doctor should remain the center of a team who work together to relieve where they cannot heal, to keep the patient's own struggle within his compass." I love that. It's the patient's compass that we have to understand—to bring hope and consolation.

Kübler-Ross says, "I say to people who care for people who are dying, 'If you really love that person and want to help them, be with them. Sit with them. You don't have to talk. You don't have to do anything. But really be there.'"

The result of all their work is that we got a federal benefit to pay for hospice. Previously, most of the hospices that grew in the United States were grassroots organizations led by volunteers from faith communities—church groups, synagogue groups. They were not part of the medical establishment in any way; they were countercultural. And they focused almost entirely on one disease: cancer—as if somehow that was what everybody died from. So the good news is that the federal benefit led to an exponential increase in access to hospice because now there was money to be made doing it; there was a way to support these programs. There are now over 5,500 hospices in the United States, 70 percent of which are for-profit. It's a big industry and rapidly growing.

Hospice has many positive effects. It lets people stay home. It has a focus on the person—the patient as a person—and their family, not just the patient. This led to very substantial improvements in quality of life and ability to remain in control of your life during a serious illness. But the weaknesses are also quite profound.

By law and by design it's only for people who have a prognosis of less than six months. Now those of you who have worked in healthcare will know that we have no idea who's going to die in six months. Absolutely no idea. Even in the cancer wing we don't know who's going to die in six months. We don't have a good sense of prognosis usually until a few weeks to maybe a month or two before death. So the design of the benefit bears no relationship to the reality of the human condition. That's the first thing.

The second thing is that people have to sign a piece of paper giving up the right of insurance coverage for treatment of their disease in order to get the hospice care. So I've had many patients say to me that it feels like they're being asked to sign their own death warrant. They're being asked to sign a piece of paper that says, *I agree I'm dying and you don't have to take care of me in the hospital any more. And in return for confessing these sins I will get hospice care.* It's quite cruel, actually, in my view, what we ask patients to do.

So hospice doesn't work for people who are not predictably and obviously dying. Alzheimer's, stroke, heart failure, emphysema, end-stage renal disease, transplant, frailty, debility: all of these are essentially inappropriate causes for hospice because we can't predict their time of death. And when hospices, to their enormous credit, tried to extend palliative care to chronically ill populations who were not dying at a predictable rate, they got slammed for fraud and abuse by the federal government and have now become extremely sensitized to that risk and much less likely to take patients who are not clearly dying.

Hospice was a piece of the solution but not the entire solution.

In the late '80s and early '90s, a bunch of private-sector philanthropists like Robert Wood Johnson and George Soros came into the business. The first thing that Johnson did was back something called the Support Study, a huge study of over nine thousand patients with serious, chronic illness. About 40 percent of these patients had spent at least ten days in an ICU in their last hospital stay, half had moderate to severe pain half the time. Between 40 and 60 percent reported moderate to severe pain after a week in the hospital, when there had been plenty of time to evaluate and respond. And over half of families experienced a major adverse impact such as bankruptcy, loss of employment, serious illness in a spouse, etc.

I want to give a few examples of what Robert Wood Johnson did then. He paid for a physician curriculum called Epic, a nursing curriculum called Ellneck, and gave David Weissman money to develop a curriculum that is available on the internet, so anyone can take it and use it to teach. They tested a whole bunch of different models of delivery of palliative care in the Promoting Excellence in End-of-Life Care project, which was led by Ira Byock. They looked at textbooks and journals and found that you could read the whole major leading medical or nursing textbook and not know that any actual people died of any of these diseases. There was no written documentation of pain or suffering or distress. It just wasn't in there—completely absent. So Robert Wood Johnson wrote to the editors and pointed out, for example, that the leading cause of death in this country is heart failure, but in the cardiology textbooks there is no death from heart failure. There is no shortness of breath, no fatigue, no depression, and no family/caregiver burden. And it changed. So now if you look at all those textbooks, they all have content in this area. And the same goes for journals. If you look at the leading journals now, they routinely carry publications on palliative care issues that were nowhere to be found ten years ago. That is really important; that is how students learn.

So that is how we got to where we are now. Thanks to these investments there are now over 1,700 hospital palliative care teams in the United States—that is the good news. The bad news is they are of highly variable quality, penetration, and impact. For instance, you can have a palliative care team if you have a full-time employee physician who only comes in after hours to do palliative care. In my view that shouldn't count, but it counts. We need to bring everyone up to a higher standard. There are new subspecialties in medicine and nursing in the last five or six years, which are highly variable and offer highly inadequate exposure to training for medical students, nursing students, social work students, chaplaincy students, and graduate education. So you should not be surprised if your doctor or your nurse knows nothing about the management of pain and nothing about how to conduct a conversation about what to expect. They probably have never been trained to do so.

We're also seeing a change in the cognitive frame for palliative care; it's moving away from brink-of-death care and away from cancer as the model toward a recognition that palliative care is good quality care for anyone with a serious illness, whether they are going to be cured, live for twenty or thirty years, or have progressive illness. It is a much broader frame of reference for palliative care than we have ever seen before.

In this new frame for palliative care, the patient receives both care focused on quality of life and whatever disease-directed therapies are appropriate; you can get treatment for both pain and disease. This would apply to someone, say a twenty-three-year-old with acute leukemia, who's going to go through hell with the diagnosis and treatment but is still going to be cured and then hopefully never see any of us again. The vast majority of patients we serve are chronically ill and living for a very long time with debilitating illnesses.

This new definition for palliative care is the one that I encourage and plead with you to use. It does not refer to prognosis. It does not say anything about dying. It doesn't say anything about giving up one kind of treatment in order to get palliative treatment. Palliative care is appropriate at any age and any stage and can be provided at the same time as curative or life-prolonging treatment.

This definition was tested with a public audience—one thousand likely voters. The Center for Advancement of Palliative Care asked them to rank what they thought were the most valuable components of palliative care. This is what we learned.

The public liked the term "specialized medical care." My nursing and social work colleagues don't like that term, but the public liked it because it's reassuring: "Oh, it's like cardiology. Oh, it's like oncology."

For people with serious illnesses, interestingly, "advanced illness" equals "terminal" in the public's eyes; they know that it's a euphemism.

They didn't like the term "suffering." We use the term all the time, but it's insider language. For the public and patients and families, the term "suffering" has a kind of death pull to it and an end-of-life pull to it, and if that's not the way the patient or the family articulate what they're going through, we should not impose that language on them. So we're learning to use words like "symptoms," "pain," and "stress," because everyone gets these.

Whatever the diagnosis, the goal is to improve quality of life for both the patient and the family. Interestingly, "patient" and "family" were the number-one identified characteristics of palliative care; they ranked higher than anything else in this definition.

Palliative care should be provided by a team. I had thought "team" would be negative; these people have enough strangers in and out of their rooms or in and out of their lives. But "team" seemed to imply "communication" to the public—that we were actually talking to each other, and they recognize that that's important, so they liked it.

Then they really liked this: work with a patient's other doctors. This is the opposite of what happens in hospice; you lose your whole team for a brand-new team at the time when you can least afford it. Instead, palliative care should be structured to provide an extra layer of support. If you're looking for an elevator pitch about what palliative care should be, it's the extra layer of support. If you've got three seconds, that's it. Everybody understands that you need an added layer of support in this broken healthcare system. Palliative shouldn't take anything away, and it shouldn't ask people to give anything up.

We took this feedback from our poll and compiled it and then brought this definition of palliative care back to the public. We deliberately chose a Republican pollster, Bill Macinturf, because we wanted to make sure this data would feel legitimate to both sides of the aisle. Bill found that the response to the definition was so positive it was embarrassing; most of his colleagues thought he made the numbers up. A very positive result in public opinion polling is in the high 60 percent range. You don't ever see public opinion in the 90 percent range. But whether you are a Tea Partier or a progressive, everybody wants palliative care when it's defined this way.

The three goals of palliative care are the relief of physical, emotional, and spiritual distress. To accomplish this really well we need expert communication about what is happening and what to expect. We need skilled coordination across all the different settings that patients traverse in a serious illness.

We actually now have a growing body of evidence that supports what we've known in our hearts to be right; the scientific evidence shows that palliative care improves quality of life, prolongs life, and markedly reduces the risk of ending up in the hospital. There are very few other interventions in the healthcare system that you could say this about.

Recently, our colleagues at Massachusetts General did an important study on newly-diagnosed lung cancer patients. The control group was given excellent cancer care only. The intervention group got excellent cancer care plus palliative care. Those who got both had better quality of life and lower rates of depression, were much less likely to be hospitalized or receive chemotherapy in the last month of life, and to everyone's surprise also lived on average 2.7 months longer.

This study hit the front page of all major media outlets. Not because of any of that other stuff, but because of those 2.7 months. My colleagues at Sinai called me and said, "Diane, did you see that paper? That can't be true!" A large number of physicians seem to believe that with palliative care you might die better, but you will also die sooner. There is no data to support that myth, but it is the firmly held cognitive frame of doctors. When I show this data to regular people, they look at me like, "What's the big deal? Of course people live longer if their quality of life is better." There's this huge disconnect between the profession and everyone else.

So what might be the mechanism of action for living longer with palliative care along with regular cancer care? What is the mechanism by which happiness might prolong life? We do know that depression is an independent predictor of mortality; if you have a stroke and are depressed, you will die sooner. If you have heart failure and are depressed, you will die sooner. If you have Alzheimer's and are depressed, you will die sooner. Depression kills, and because there was a lot less depression in the palliative care group, they lived longer.

Okay, what about symptom control? Why would that help someone live longer? Pain also kills, and shortness of breath also kills. Perhaps they're so stressful that all of your body's energy and focus goes into bearing them, which takes away your resources from other things. It's not clear, but that's a second possibility. What else?

Personal human connection. What might be the mechanism of action of that? There is an increasing body of evidence suggesting that mood impacts the immune system. Some people still reject it as too "touchy feely," but I showed this data at a talk at a medical school in Cincinnati, and for some reason there were scientists in the audience, which is unusual, and one of them stood up in the back and said, "There was a study of mice who had received transplants and were immune-system suppressed, and some mice were randomly assigned to have great care but be alone. They had clean cages but were in the cages by themselves. They had food when they were supposed to get food, but that was it. The other group was randomly assigned to a much more interesting environment where there were a lot more shavings and pieces of cloth and toys. There was also more handling and talking from the staff, and access to food and other mice. This group lived four times longer than the control group." So basically the biggest impact on survival wasn't made by the drugs; it was all the stuff that everyone in the real world understands is so critical to general well-being.

And finally, what do we know about being in the hospital if you are sick? It's dangerous. It's really dangerous. If you don't absolutely have to be there, you should get out. And the reason is not that people there aren't trying hard, not that they don't care about you, not that they aren't doing their best—it's the risk of error, the risk of serious infection, the risk of falling in a strange place or becoming confused in a strange place, the risk of having your meds mixed up. There are over one hundred thousand deaths per year in this country that occur because someone was in the hospital. If you are a lung cancer patient and you are immune-suppressed with chemotherapy and radiation and you get a C. diff infection, you die. The risk to more vulnerable populations is even higher. So avoiding the hospital is actually among the most powerful explanations for this gain in life expectancy. This is really hard to get across to the public; people persist in believing the hospital is the one safe place. We have to figure out a way to change that cognitive frame among the public.

We live in a society in which the quality of medical care is among the poorest on the globe. We rank fortieth in quality of disease treatment among other nations, fortieth in infant and maternal mortality, fortieth in preventable mortality. As I said, there are one hundred thousand deaths per year in hospitals for preventable medical errors. One-seventh of our population is uninsured and has no access to healthcare, and healthcare is the number-one cause of bankruptcy in this country. In no other developed nation is that the case. Healthcare is the number-one cause of the decline in American society because we are spending almost one-fifth of our economy on it at this point.

Palliative care is central to the nation's future because we take care of the sickest and most complex patients—who also happen to account for 50 percent of all healthcare spending. So we are sitting right at the center of the bull's-eye. Our patient population is the most vulnerable to poor quality care and is the most expensive. Who do you think is going to get targeted in financial cuts? Our patient population. As it happens, we improve their quality of life while reducing their costs. So palliative care is the solution here. We have got to stop seeing ourselves as marginalized and unimportant and start seeing ourselves as the center of the future of the healthcare system.

Here's an example. My colleague David Casserat had a patient, a seventy-nine-year-old woman, admitted through the emergency department for management of pain due to metastatic lung cancer. Her pain was eight out of ten, on admission of which she was taking Tylenol. She had been admitted four times within six months: twice for pain, once for nausea and dehydration, and once for altered mental status. Her eighty-seven-year-old husband was overwhelmed. She said, "I told the doctor that I never wanted to go back to the hospital. It's torture. I have no control and can't do anything for myself, and I get weaker and sicker. Every time I'm in the hospital, it feels like I will never get out." And her husband: "She hates being in the hospital, but what could I do? The pain was terrible, and I couldn't reach the oncologist." This oncologist actually had "If this is an emergency, call 911" on the tape, so that is exactly what they did. "I couldn't even move her myself, so I called the ambulance. It was the only thing I could do." Now this patient eventually got into a home palliative care program where she lived another six months, continuing to get chemotherapy, and then got hospice through the last month of her life after that.

So these are the challenges for patients and families: no coordination, lack of support, no attention to goals or preferences, poor symptom management. But what about the healthcare systems in which they get care? Their care is very costly, they are frequently put in the most expensive setting, and they hate being there, like the woman in the example above.

Right now, thanks to healthcare reform, hospitals are actually being financially penalized for frequent readmissions and deaths. So all of a sudden, we have leverage because we can now help hospitals avoid those penalties by helping people stay safer at home.

It's not enough to have access to palliative care in hospitals, which is where we've got it now. Most illness occurs at home and in communities. We need home palliative care regardless of prognosis or goals. It shouldn't matter how long you're going to live; it should matter what your need is. And so the next stage of development is to ensure access to palliative care across all settings, across all stages of illness, no matter where you live, no matter what color you are, no matter hold old you are.

We must increase public awareness of palliative care so people start demanding it. Demanding it of policy makers, demanding it of the providers. We have to educate patients, families, and providers. This is one of the goals of the New York Zen Center for Contemplative Care.

We also have to get to a point where healthcare professionals have the knowledge and skills to provide this kind of contemplative care.

Most of my colleagues do not know how to identify whether or not someone is dying. They send their patients to the ICU because they're getting worse. They literally don't recognize the dying process because they have not been taught to do so.

Why are things so bad? Medical students, residents, and fellows get virtually no exposure to good contemplative care practice or good palliative care practice during serious illness. "Ah, Mr. Bromley, nice to put a face on a disease." That is how we are taught. We are taught to say, "It is the lung cancer patient in bed three." It is more about the disease than it is about the person; that's what you get when you are a patient.

We have to train more people in contemplative palliative care. We've got to make it easier for people in the middle of their career to be able to get contemplative training and enter the field. And we have to make sure that currently practicing doctors and nurses and those being trained all have core competencies in palliative care. We can't depend on specialists to take care of this.

Palliative care has a procedure. Even though we don't do colonoscopy or angioplasty or infused chemotherapy or operate on people, which is how you get paid in the healthcare profession, we have a critical procedure. I think everybody who is engaged in contemplative approaches to care understands just how hard it is. It is rocket science. It is brain surgery. It's hard, and it takes training. It takes training and practice and that is what everyone in the medical field needs to get.

I have a question I ask a lot, once I've gotten to know a patient or family: "How are you feeling inside yourself?" I keep a journal of the responses. One of my patients was a woman who was the center of her church and the center of her extended family, and she had breast cancer that was so advanced when she came in, because she hated doctors and hated hospitals, that there was very little we could do medically to prolong her life. But this is what she said in answer to that question: "I am talking to God. I don't think I can take this pain anymore. I am so worried about my family. I wish I could get away from all this. I am not sure how my husband will manage without me. I want to go home. I am at peace." I have never had somebody say to me, "I want to be cured." I have never had somebody say to me, "I am terrified of dying." When you are where the person is, you can be present with them in that place. But you have to ask the right question. If your question is "How is your pain on a scale of zero to ten?" then you will only get a number.

There is not only patient suffering; there is—very importantly—professional suffering. I want to tell you about Judy Friedman, who was a patient of mine a few years ago. She was sixty-five years old, diagnosed with cancer at age fifty-nine, no smoking history, initially given a prognosis of about a year, lived six years partly because she was just lucky, partly because she had a great oncologist whom she was devoted to and adored. I met her about two years before she would die. She found me on the internet and came to see me because she recognized that her oncologist was unable to talk to her about what might happen if the treatment stopped working, and she was somebody who wanted to know. She wanted control. So her oncologist and I comanaged her for the last two years of her life, and I worked on things like fatigue, pain, and talking to her daughter and her husband. When her disease started progressing in spite of everything that the oncologist had tried, she went to hospice for only three weeks and died very peacefully at home.

When Judy's brain metastases were progressing, she had headaches and difficulty concentrating. Her oncologist offered her the placement of a reservoir in her brain to give what's called intrathecal chemotherapy directly into the metastatic lesions of the brain. Judy came to see me, and the conversation we had was the most profound learning experience of my career—and maybe my entire life so far. She said, "Dr. C said I should have intrathecal chemotherapy. What do you think?" I am old enough by now to suppress the urge to say, "That's absolutely ridiculous! What is he talking about?" Instead I said, "You know, Judy, I don't know. This is not my area of expertise, but I'll call him and we'll talk about it and one of us will get back to you." So I called him and I said, "You know, Dr. C, Judy was in to see me today. She said that you had recommended intrathecal chemotherapy. I don't have much experience with this procedure. What are you hoping we can accomplish for her?" Doing my best to be completely without judgment and open, right? He said, "It won't help her." So I had to swallow my own opinions and my own cause—with self-awareness, self-knowledge, I can know that what I am feeling is not always what I should act on. There was a long pause, and so I did the Judo thing. I reversed my impulse and said, "Do you want me to encourage her to go ahead with it?" And here is what he said: "I don't want Judy to think I am abandoning her."

Do you see why this was such a profound moment for me? It completely shifted my perspective on why sometimes my colleagues do things that make absolutely no sense to me at all. This doctor loved Judy, was totally devoted to her, had performed magic in order to keep her going for a really long time. He had no more oncology treatments to offer her and no other means of expressing his love for her. So he offered her a futile treatment because it was the only arrow in his quiver. So as soon as he said that—and this is the power of self-awareness and naming feelings—as soon as he said, "I don't want Judy to think I am abandoning her," he then immediately followed with "We are not going to do that." Right away. *Because he wasn't conscious of his behavior until I asked the question, and he answered it.*

Practice asking the right question. Being there. Ask questions instead of telling people what to do.

After that, Judy was home on hospice. On one of my visits there I asked how she was feeling inside herself, and she said, "I am really angry at Dr. C. He has not called, and he has not come to see me." And it is so interesting that her whole inner-life was trying to understand this experience of betrayal by this doctor whom she was devoted to and adored. It was not being spent on her parents, her husband, her daughter, or her book group. It was about her doctor, her feeling of betrayal by the doctor. "Why isn't he coming to see me, why hasn't he called?" After a conversation, she agreed to let me call him. "You know, Dr. C," I said. "Judy really wants to see you." And he said, "Why? I can't help her." He still felt that the only thing he had to offer was cancer treatment. I said, "Actually she wants to thank you and she wants to say goodbye. She really loves you." He went and made his first home visit. After he saw her, she was a different person—much more peaceful and more able to be present. Education is critical for all of us.

All hospitals, nursing homes, home care agencies, and doctors' offices should have the capacity to deliver this kind of care, and the model should be that we have hospice services inpatient units, outpatient clinics, cancer center palliative care, outpatient primary care clinics, nursing home service, and home care. This is the vision: Wherever you go, there is palliative care. You shouldn't have to be in the hospital or be in hospice—palliative care can be just part of what you get when you have a serious illness. Isaac Eisenoff said, "Life is pleasant, death is peaceful. It's the transition that is troublesome." That's what we are here for. I love these words from William Gibson: "The future is here now, it is just not evenly distributed." So that is why our work is so important, so that care becomes evenly distributed.

Contemplative care is the embodiment, ethos, and practice of palliative care. It *is* palliative care. And those of us who are not Buddhist monks are borrowing from the wisdom traditions to practice the work that we do with patients. Contemplative care is a coming home. Thank you, reader, for your work and efforts on behalf of all of us.

Watch with Me: The Founding of St. Christopher's Hospice

2

Dame Cicely Saunders

We can think about the foundations of St. Christopher's in various ways. We can say that the foundations are made up of all the interest and the money that has been given and promised and that has made the building and the laying of the foundation stone possible. We can think about them as all the work that has ever been done in this field in the past by people other than ourselves and on which we will build our own work. We can think about them as the people who have gradually joined in thinking, praying, and working for St. Christopher's ever since the vision was first given more than seventeen years ago. I like best of all to think of St. Christopher's as being founded on patients, those we have known and who are now safely through this part of their lives.

Now I want to look at our foundations by looking at one particular phrase that I believe expresses the ideals of St. Christopher's—the summing up of all the needs of the dying that was made for us in the Garden of Gethsemane—the simple words "watch with me." I think the one word "watch" says many things on many different levels, all of importance to us. In the first place, it demands that all the work at St. Christopher's should stem from respect for the patient and very close attention to his distress. It means really looking at him, learning what this kind of pain is like, what these symptoms are like, and from this knowledge finding out how best to relieve them. It means continually gaining new skills, developing those already learned from teachers and institutions and from discussion with many other people. I have not found any individual place concentrating on these problems alone, but many have helped to shed light on different facets of them, and all this we want to bring together and develop into new skills in an area that is very greatly neglected.

Not Only Skill but Compassion Also

We want to plan and carry out research in the relief of distress such as has not been done anywhere else, so far as I have been able to discover. It is often easier in a specialist setting to go on learning in this way. By building what we think is an ideal unit, we hope to be able to help not only our own patients, but to raise standards generally and also to stimulate others to think about these problems. A patient comes to my mind here, a young woman who said, "You seem to understand the pain from *both* sides." Our aim in learning is to give the kind of relief described by another woman who said, "It was *all* pain, but now it's gone and I am free."

Seventeen years ago, a young Pole died and left me £500 to be "a window in your Home." This was the very beginning of St. Christopher's. I also remember him saying, "I only want what is in your mind and in your heart." This was echoed years later by another Pole who said to us, "Thank you. And not just for your pills but for your heart." I think both of them showed that they wanted not only skill but compassion also. They needed warmth and friendship as well as good technical care. I think our understanding of what real "watching" means must include this.

We have, indeed, to learn what this pain is like. Still more, we have to learn what it feels like to be so ill, to be leaving life and its activity, to know that your faculties are failing, that you are parting from loves and responsibilities. We have to learn how to feel "with" patients without feeling "like" them if we are to give the kind of listening and steady support that they need to find their own way through.

Here again comes a key phrase I have often quoted: "I look for someone to look as if they are trying to understand me." These patients are not looking for pity and indulgence but for us to look at them with respect and an expectation of courage, a heritage from seeing people like the woman who said to me, "You can tell them all that it was *all right*." She was not going through a strange, dramatic, or just unlucky experience, to be written up as such with sentimentality or sensationalism, but an all-too-common experience such as ordinary people have always faced and somehow managed to come through.

Following Their Path

We will be seeing patients who go along the path that leads from the honest but wistful plea "I do not *want* to die, I do not *want* to die" to the quiet acceptance of "I only want what is right." We will not only see acceptance but also a very real joy, the true gaiety of someone who has gone through doubt, fear, and unwillingness and come out the other side. I remember coming away from the bedside of a man who had come along that difficult path just about an hour before he died and saying to myself—"He looked *amused*"—and he really did. Certainly we are going to see hard things, but we are also going to see rewards and compensations and insight given to our patients here and now, and we will see an extraordinary amount of real happiness and even light-heartedness.

Planning an ideal unit is not enough to interpret all the meanings of the word "watch" if teaching is not a vital part of what we do. We want St. Christopher's to be a place where all kinds of people can join us to learn from our experience and learn from our patients with us. This does not mean burdening the patients with the demands of continual bedside teaching. It does mean that you can give them an interest I know they enjoy if it is done in the right way. It can also reveal a new purpose in what is happening to them and what they are doing themselves. Certainly they are not all going to be saints. Some will be, indeed, and we will be very honored and helped by their coming to us. Others will be splendidly maddening, and I have no time to suggest the various crises with which we are going to have to cope. But who is to say who does the best—the person whose last weeks are the crown of a life of devotion, the young girl who makes the whole ward into a party for months on end and never shows you how much it costs her, or the old man who just manages to stop grumbling for his last ten days or so? Certainly we will never fail to learn from them, and some of the things that we will learn may surprise our future staff. Work here will not just be solemn. Rather, I would just say it will be real, and reality is gay and funny as well as serious. Above all, it will never be dull.

Being There

"Watch with me" means still more than our attempts to understand mental suffering and loneliness and to pass on what we have learned. It means also a great deal that cannot be understood. Those words did not mean "understand what is happening" when they were first spoken. Still less did they mean "explain" or "take away." However much we can ease distress, however much we can help the patients to find a new meaning in what is happening, there will always be the place where we will have to stop and know that we are really helpless. It would be very wrong indeed if, at that point, we tried to forget that this was so and to pass by. It would be wrong if we tried to cover it up, to deny it, and to delude ourselves that we were always successful. Even when we feel that we can do absolutely nothing, we will still have to be prepared to stay.

"Watch with me" means, above all, just "be there." I remember the patient who said of the people who had really helped her, "They never let you down. They just keep on coming." I also remember she described the way God had met her: "He sends me people." I am quite certain that St. Christopher's has to learn to be a place where people do not let you down but instead give the feeling of reassurance and safety that comes from faithfulness.

I think this need especially stems from the demand that we should grow into a real community. It is very important that we should be a group of people who have confidence in each other, that St. Christopher's should be the kind of family and home that can give the welcome and hospitality of a good home, where people are accepted as themselves and can relax in security. It must also be a place where everyone knows that individual contributions matter and that there is no hierarchy of importance in what is done. Who will know what or who matters most to an individual patient as his manifold problems are dealt with by various members of such a group? There is a kind of compassionate matter-of-factness that develops in such a place, and in this the hard-pressed worker is not overwhelmed by her own responsibilities.

The Community of All People

Above all, I think that it is here that we see the very great need for a religious foundation. We must remember that we belong to the much wider community of the whole church, to the whole communion of saints and, indeed, to the whole community of all men. It is because of this that St. Christopher's is ecumenical and nondenominational. We will welcome people of all sorts and kinds and be of all sorts and kinds ourselves. We are not emphasizing that there is just one way, but rather that there is one Person coming in many ways.

The same words "Watch with me" remind us also that we have not begun to see their meaning until we have some awareness of Christ's presence both in the patient and in the watcher. We will remember his oneness with all sufferers, for that is true for all time whether they recognize it here or not. As we watch, we know that he has been here, that he still is here, and that his presence is redemptive.

Through Symbols and Sacraments

Christ will be present in all the skills that we learn and in symbols and sacraments of all kinds. These will include the sacraments of the cup of cold water and the washing of the disciples' feet. All these things will speak silently to the patients about God's love for them. So, too, will the whole planning and decoration of the building itself, thought out over a very long period with our architect and carried out by him with great insight and imagination. Especially, I think, it will be shown in the planning of the chapel and in all the pictures, the symbols, and the sculptures that are being created by artists who share this faith with us. It is very important that this message should be shown in these different ways. I have seen again and again how receptive patients are to the things they look at when they are not able to bear talking any longer. Often it is important that very little should be said at all because it is so easy to interrupt a real message.

So much of our communication with people is done without words, but I think this is especially so with the very ill. The patient who says soon after her admission, "It is marvelous to begin to feel safe again," has been met by the atmosphere and by the things she looks at just as much as by the nursing and by the drugs and relief she is given. In a whole climate of safety she finds her own key and her own meeting. We will see patients able to listen, perhaps for the first time, to something that has been said to them all their lives, but for which they have somehow never had time for real attention.

I have been impressed again and again by the way patients will lie and look at a picture or a crucifix and how much these can say to them. I believe that it is very important that these should be works created now, by artists who are interpreting these truths in the context of the world today.

"My Bags Are Packed . . ."

Remember the words of Pope John when he said, "My bags are packed, and I can leave with a tranquil heart at any moment." I think that this is how we pray for all the patients who come to us. We remember that some of them are already ill, frail, lonely, or despairing, and we pray for them. Others are busy and have no thought of calamity. Perhaps only in calamity are they going to find the meaning of the whole of the rest of their lives. I think that we should pray that we will be able to make it possible for them to pack their bags with the right things, pack them with what matters, with what *they* need—that while they are here they will find all that they need for reconciliation, fulfillment, and meaning as they go through this last part of their lives.

To Be Silent, to Listen, to Be There

I have tried to sum up the demands of this work we are planning in the words "Watch with me." Our most important foundation for St. Christopher's is the hope that in watching we should learn not only how to free patients from pain and distress, how to understand them and never let them down, but also how to be silent, how to listen, and how just to be there. As we learn this, we will also learn that the real work is not ours at all. We are building for so much more than ourselves. I think if we try to remember this we will see that the work is truly to the greater glory of God.

The Promise

Marie Howe

In the dream I had when he came back not sick
but whole, and wearing his winter coat,

he looked at me as though he couldn't speak, as if
there were a law against it, a membrane he couldn't break.

His silence was what he could not
not do, like our breathing in this world, like our living,

as we do, in time.
And I told him: I'm reading all this Buddhist stuff,

and listen, we don't die when we die. Death is an event,
a threshold we pass through. We go on and on

and into light forever.
And he looked down, and then back up at me. It was the look
we'd pass

across the table when Dad was drunk again and dangerous,
the level look that wants to tell you something,
in a crowded room, something important, and can't.

The Gate

Marie Howe

I had no idea that the gate I would step through
to finally enter this world

would be the space my brother's body made. He was
a little taller than me: a young man

but grown, himself by then,
done at twenty-eight, having folded every sheet,

rinsed every glass he would ever rinse under the cold
and running water.

This is what you have been waiting for, he used to say to me.
And I'd say, What?

And he'd say, This—holding up my cheese and mustard sandwich.
And I'd say, What?

And he'd say, This, sort of looking around.

For Three Days

Marie Howe

For three days now I've been trying to think of another word
  for gratitude
because my brother could have died and didn't,

because for a week we stood in the intensive care unit trying
  not to imagine
how it would be then, afterwards.

My youngest brother, Andy, said: This is so weird. I don't know
  if I'll be
talking with John today, or buying a pair of pants for his funeral.

And I hated him for saying it because it was true and seemed
  to tilt it,
because I had been writing his elegy in my head during the
  seven-hour drive there

and trying not to. Thinking meant not thinking. It meant
  imagining my brother
surrounded by light—like Schrödinger's Cat that would be dead
  if you looked

and might live if you didn't. And then it got better, and then it
  got worse.
And it's a story now: He came back.

And I did, by that time, imagine him dead. And I did begin to
write the other story:
how the crowd in the stifling church snapped to a tearful
attention,

how my brother lived again, for a few minutes, through me.
And although I know I couldn't help it, because fear has its own
language

and its own story, because even grief provides a living remedy,
I can't help but think of that woman who said to him whom she
considered

her savior: If thou hadst been here my brother had not died,
how she might
have practiced her speech, and how she too might have stood
trembling,

unable to meet the eyes of the dear familiar figure that stumbled
from the cave,
when the compassionate fist of God opened and crushed her with
gratitude and shame.

The Last Time

Marie Howe

The last time we had dinner together in a restaurant
with white tablecloths, he leaned forward

and took my two hands in his hands and said,
I'm going to die soon. I want you to know that.

And I said, I think I do know.
And he said, What surprises me is that you don't.

And I said, I do. And he said, What?
And I said, Know that you're going to die.

And he said, No, I mean know that you are.

What the Living Do

Marie Howe

Johnny, the kitchen sink has been clogged for days,
some utensil probably fell down there.
And the Drano won't work but smells dangerous, and the
crusty dishes have piled up

waiting for the plumber I still haven't called. This is the
everyday we spoke of.
It's winter again: the sky's a deep headstrong blue, and the
sunlight pours through

the open living-room windows because the heat's on too high
in here, and I can't turn it off.
For weeks now, driving, or dropping a bag of groceries in the
street, the bag breaking,

I've been thinking: This is what the living do. And yesterday,
hurrying along those
wobbly bricks in the Cambridge sidewalk, spilling my coffee
down my wrist and sleeve,

I thought it again, and again later, when buying a hairbrush:
This is it.
Parking. Slamming the car door shut in the cold. What you
called that yearning.

What you finally gave up. We want the spring to come and the
winter to pass. We want

whoever to call or not call, a letter, a kiss—we want more and
    more and then more of it.

But there are moments, walking, when I catch a glimpse of
    myself in the window glass,
say, the window of the corner video store, and I'm gripped by a
    cherishing so deep

for my own blowing hair, chapped face, and unbuttoned coat
    that I'm speechless:
I am living, I remember you.

Mindfulness Is Not a Part-Time Job: Dementia, Flowers, and Attention

3

Issan Dorsey

I was talking with a friend recently about the phrase "coming to reside in your breath-mind," and working with the phrase, and how useful it has been to me. I thought it was interesting that I'd never really heard it before and was just now beginning to work with it.

We have to be willing to explore and experiment in our practice. To do this, we have to have a sense of humor and a willingness to explore and experiment with our lives and our uncomfortableness. For instance, we know that sometimes we can sit for a few minutes, or even a few days, and at some point it gets pretty uncomfortable.

Lately I have been exploring this way of thinking with a friend who has AIDS dementia; the virus is living in his brain. I'm thinking and working on it and talking with him about it because the virus that is attacking so many of us now ends up being in the brain. So is there some way for us, who aren't sick, to experience that with him? I don't know yet. My question is this: How can we be with people who have dementia? And how can we experience the dementia—delusion—that we all have anyway? Mind is always creating confusion, joy, depression, "like," and "don't like." But there is also a "background mind." This background mind is what my friend and I have been discussing.

Sometimes when I'm talking about uncomfortableness, I talk about the five fears—fear of dying, fear of illness, fear of dementia, fear of loss of livelihood, and fear of public speaking. Especially the third one: the fear of unusual states of mind. How can we come to have appreciation and respect for this fear and not just resistance, so that we can enter our fear, allowing these new areas of uncomfortableness? When we can enter each of these new spaces, we can begin to look at truthfulness.

Why do we have to sit? Really, if we're completely sincere, then there's no reason to sit. I'm not completely sincere, so I have to keep sitting to check on myself. Even if we're involved with unskillful actions, the one quality we should strive for is truthfulness. Truthfulness takes a total commitment to see all aspects of ourselves and our unskillfulness. Then, if we can embrace the totality of ourselves, we can embrace the totality of others and of the world. Even when we see a beautiful flower, we say, "Oh what a beautiful flower." "Beautiful flower" is extra. Just look at the flower.

Suzuki Roshi wrote, "When we practice zazen, our mind is calm and quite simple. But usually our mind is very busy and complicated, and it is difficult to be concentrating on what we are doing." This is because when we act, we think, and this thinking leaves some trace. Our activity is shadowed by some preconceived idea. The traces and notions make our mind very complicated. When we do something with a simple, clear mind, we have no shadows and our activity is strong and straightforward.

Even zazen practice gets so complicated. We're dissecting every aspect of what's going on, reviewing and comparing. How do we keep it simple and straightforward? How do we come to know this basic truth of practice and Buddhism? The teaching and the rules can and should change according to the situation and the people we're practicing with, but the secret of practice cannot be changed. It's always truth.

We teach ourselves and encourage ourselves by creating this space, the meditation hall, so we can begin looking at our minds. "Don't invite your thoughts to tea" is an expression of Suzuki Roshi's that I've always found useful. Now I'm saying, "*Create* background mind."

This practice is simple: watch your breaths and don't invite your thoughts to tea. But not inviting your thoughts to tea doesn't mean to get rid of thinking. That is discrimination. So there's no reason to get rid of thoughts, but rather to have a blank, noninterfering relationship with them. Don't make your mind blank, but rather have some blank relationship with the thoughts. Begin to see the space behind and around the thoughts. Shift the seat of your identity out of your thoughts and come to reside in your breath-mind. We develop our intention to reside in our breath-mind by first bringing our intention to "breath as mind," and then by shifting the seat of our identity from our thoughts to our breath.

This all ties in with how we use the meditation hall, this laboratory. We should have a willingness to explore with our lives, and this is our laboratory right here—how we use the meditation hall and how we use what happens outside of it. Mindfulness is not a part-time job.

Unfinished Business and How You Know That You Know

4

Elisabeth Kübler-Ross

We are here to talk about death and dying, and the first thing I want to share with you is that if you need something all you really need to do is ask and it will be given to you. It will not always be what you think you want, but it will always be given.

In the last twelve years my whole life has been like this. If we would listen to dying patients and all the things they begin to open to, we'd find that they are very willing to share the things they learn with those who have a longer time to live, even though it is usually too late for them in their own lives. Dying patients are the best teachers in the whole wide world, and they teach you not only about the process of dying, which is very easy to understand, but also about the process of living. To live fully means not being afraid of living and not being afraid of dying.

I was born an unwanted child to parents who very much wanted a baby. They were expecting a very chubby and rosy nine-pound beauty. What they got was a very ugly two-pound shrimp. After fifteen minutes another two-pounder came, and that was the answer to my ugly two pounds. A half hour later, a third baby girl was born.

I don't know whether any of you have been raised as a triplet, but I wouldn't wish it on my enemy. Fifty-five years ago it was very rare to have triplets; today it is far more common. Our parents dressed all of us alike. We had the same bedclothes, the same bedspreads, the same teachers, the same grade cards. No matter how miserable or how excellent I was in school, it never really mattered because the teacher didn't know who anyone was anyway. They just gave each of us a "C."

You think it's funny, but for children it was really tragic because no matter what we did it was like no one really cared. We each wanted to be outstanding or terrible at something just to have an identity. My sister's earliest memory was when my father gave her a bath twice and skipped me. Nobody knew who was who.

My one sister was always on my mother's lap, and my other sister was always on my father's lap. There was no third lap, and I was too arrogant and defiant to ask, "When is it my turn? I need a lap, too." So I got close to bunnies, to animals, to nature. I became interconnected with nature but isolated from interpersonal relationships, short of the superficial family meals and trips together. I never shared how lonely and isolated I was.

We were very well to do—an upper-middle-class family, a gorgeous house, beautiful gardens, and beautiful dresses. And I hated all of it because no one knew I existed, really; no one knew whether I was me or my sister or my other sister. And this upbringing was the biggest, biggest, biggest blessing in my life. I learned at a very young age that regardless of all the material things and goodies you may have, if you don't have people who know who you are as a human being, you have nothing.

When I came to the United States and began my work with dying patients, I began to realize that not only dying patients teach us about the stages of grief—so does every human being who faces a loss. A little child who loses his security blanket because the mother decides it's too dirty and throws it away. Or maybe you plant a tree, and in the winter it freezes. Or your house burns down, or you lose somebody through separation or divorce or through suicide or murder. Or maybe you lose your ability to walk, your vision, your hearing, or sometimes even just a contact lens—you go through the stages of dying. You understand, this process has nothing specifically to do with dying.

People who think they're doing their children a service by protecting them need to look more closely. Should you shield the canyon from the wind storm? If you did, you would never see the beauty of its carvings.

If you see your children making a mistake or on the verge of making a mistake, let them. Let them fall. Let them cry. Let them share their pain. But also, let them share their incredible pride when no one comes and picks them up the moment they fall. Because that develops incredible self-worth—that feeling of "By golly, I can make it on my own two feet." Their lives may be full of storms, but they will also be full of the beautiful carvings that you only get if you are exposed to all the winds of life.

If someone is raised in a greenhouse where everything is nice and smooth, they become very dull and boring, and they will never, ever be able to say, "My life was beautiful." Instead they will say what 90 percent of my adult patients have said: "I made a living, but I never really lived." Your life is your free choice. You must see this.

When you work with dying patients, do not come with emotional support and your ideas about the stages of dying, being spiritual and all that stuff. First and foremost you have to take care of a patient's physical needs. A patient who is climbing the walls in pain cannot hear a pastor. A patient who is itching and being driven crazy has no use for spiritual guidance. A patient who gets pain shots that make him dopey cannot communicate or work on unfinished business. So what you need to do for terminal patients is to keep them dry and totally hydrated and pain free. First take care of all the physical needs, then take care of all the emotional needs—the unfinished business.

What fears do you have? You can name a million. But there are only two natural fears—God-given to help us survive. One is fear of high places; if you put a child on a high cliff, he will never jump off. The other is fear of loud noises. Right now, if a loud noise—a gun—were to go off behind me, I would run for my life. Those fears are natural gifts to help preserve life. All other fears keep you from living. They all result from unfinished business.

Everything natural gives us energy and helps us to fulfill our lives. Grief is a natural emotion, a gift to help you come to grips with the reality of loss. When children hurt themselves, they cry. If they are told, especially boys, not to cry, they end up with unshed tears. Just go to a movie theater and see the tears; it is the only socially acceptable place to cry. Even there, just before the lights go on, everyone takes a tissue and wipes up their tears. Why are we so ashamed to cry? It is a God-given gift to cry. If you force yourself not to cry, natural grief will turn to unnatural self-pity. It is one of the biggest tragedies of our lives. You have no idea.

Anger is a beautiful gift, and it is over in fifteen seconds if it is allowed to be natural. You are allowed to say "No thank you" if your mother wants to tie your shoes and you are twelve years old. Do you understand? You can say, "No. Thank you." That is natural, beautiful anger that makes you healthy and strong. If people are punished for acting naturally and honestly they become full of the unnatural anger and hate that fills our prisons.

Jealousy is a beautiful trait—to be jealous of someone who can read better than you is a beautiful thing. This kind of challenge develops the intellectual part of us, inspiring children to learn to emulate one another and keep working toward excellence.

Love is actually the biggest problem. We need love, of course, but there is also confused love: for instance, the mother and the shoelace. Love must be able to say no.

Nine-year-old Jeffrey spent most of his life in the hospital. He had every treatment that you can imagine. Then a young physician came to the hospital and said, "We are going to start another experimental chemotherapy." The mother and father were so depleted; no one spoke up. I happened to be visiting that day, and I said, "Has anyone asked Jeffrey what he wants?" And everyone said no. And I said, "You have to ask Jeffrey because if Jeffrey fights against another round of chemotherapy, he will die getting the therapy. But if he really wants another year or another few months of life, he will fight along with you and will have a good chance."

They asked Jeffrey, and he looked up at all of us in disgust. "I don't know why you have to make us kids so sick in order to make us well."

It was a very clear "no thank you." And his parents were able to hear this because they loved him enough. They were able to say, "Would you like us to take you home?" And Jeffrey said, "Yes." I was ready to say goodbye then, but he said, "No, you will come with me." I looked at my watch because I have a lot of Jeffreys, but he said, "It won't take long." So I said to him, "Do we have some unfinished business?" And he said, "Yes!"

We drove to suburbia, into the driveway, and into the garage. Jeffrey said, "I want Dad to take my bicycle down from the wall." It was three years old but brand new. It was Jeffrey's biggest dream to ride his bike around the block, but he was too sick to ever do it. "Dad," he said. "I want you to put the training wheels on." I don't know whether you know how painful it is for a nine-year-old to have training wheels put on. I can't tell you just how sick this child was—pale, weak. He looked at me and said, while holding the bike up, "And you, all you need to do is hold my mom back."

His mother had never learned to hold herself back, to not prop him up, and she'd cheated him of his greatest victories. So I'm holding on to the mom, and the father is holding on to me, all while this very sick child climbs onto the bicycle and takes off. He rides around the block and comes back with a huge, beaming grin across his face, and with the same authoritarian voice says, "Dad, you can take the training wheels off, shine up the bike, and carry it up to my room. When Dougie comes home from first grade send him up." Two weeks later Dougie, the next youngest, told us what had happened upstairs. Jeffrey had told him he wanted him to have his bicycle as a gift for his birthday, which was two weeks later. "I won't be around at your birthday," Jeffrey had said. But it wasn't an unconditional gift. It was given with one condition: "Never ever ever use those damn training wheels."

This work is not intrinsically depressing. It's only depressing when we impose our own needs, our own patterns, and we don't know when to call it quits. If we had given this child the experimental chemotherapy—and that was a real possibility—those parents would never have gotten to see Jeffrey ride around the block on that bicycle.

Unconditional love means that I hear you and I respect your own free choice. When you spend time with dying children, you see that very young children cannot verbalize requests, but they can communicate through spontaneous drawings. All human beings—if they speak a foreign language, if they are on a machine and they can't speak anymore, if they've had a stroke and they can't speak anymore—all you need to give them is a piece of paper and a box of crayons and ask them to spontaneously draw a picture. Grown-ups take ten minutes because they think they have to impress you. Children are honest; they take five minutes. Children—five years old—will tell you their inner understanding of their impending death. They will, through their drawings, show you what unfinished business they have. You can hear them. You can read their pictures and learn exactly the nature of the help they need and from whom it should come.

A physician came to my workshop, and we challenged him about the treatment of his cancer patients. We told him about the drawings. He said that he wanted to learn more, so we told him, "When you have a patient with a diagnosis of cancer, simply ask them to draw a picture. If you have a patient for whom you might consider chemotherapy, or radial therapy, or surgery, ask them to draw a picture, and you will know within ten minutes which of these treatments will make them well." After a year, his surgeries had been reduced by 50 percent and his patients were getting amazingly well.

He had a middle-aged man diagnosed with cancer. The doctor asked the man to conceive of his cancer. The man drew a man with a big, fat belly full of red concentric circles. That is how he visualized his cancer. Then we asked him to conceive of the chemotherapy, which from our perspective was absolutely the treatment of choice. The patient drew black arrows hitting every cancer cell, but getting deflected away rather than penetrating them.

Now, would you want to put this man on chemotherapy? And, as it turned out, not one of the chemotherapies effectively touched the cancer. From a purely intellectual point of view, this made absolutely no sense.

We asked him, "What did the doctor tell you about the chemotherapy?" And the man said, "The doctor says the chemotherapy kills the cancer cells." I was ready to say, "Yes, what are you waiting for?" He very apologetically looked at me and said, "'Thou shalt not kill.'" He went on to say that he was a Quaker. Now, I'm not a Quaker and so I said, "Not even your own cancer cells?" "No," he said. "I truly believe that 'Thou shalt not kill.'"

Unconditional love practiced in everyday life means loving my neighbor and respecting my neighbor from where he is coming from, not where I want him to be. So I said to him, "This world would be a better place if people truly did believe in 'Thou shalt not kill' and live that way." Now that he was not feeling criticized, I said to him, "You understand I have needs, too. I want you to get well, so do me a favor. Go home and conceive of how you can get well. That is *my* need."

A week later, same man, same treating physician, everything the same. I said, "Did you conceive how you could get rid of your cancer?" He drew the most gorgeous picture I have ever seen. In his picture every cancer cell is full of gnomes—those little guys with hoods. The whole belly was full of them, carrying every cancer cell away. This man was put on chemotherapy and is well today.

Do you understand the beauty in holistic medicine? Holistic medicine does not mean to throw the baby out with the bath water, to throw everything good out that we have created, but instead to take the best of traditional medicine and the best of the healing arts and simply acknowledge that every human being consists of a physical, intellectual, emotional, and spiritual quadrant. We must accept that reality and take care of all of it, not by telling the patient that he must do something and get mad at him if he doesn't, but to let him teach me and I teach him. Then we can both benefit.

I lecture all over the world, and sometimes it gets very boring. I speak to about fifteen thousand people a week from Egypt to Jerusalem to Alaska to Maui, and I say the same thing over and over. But something keeps me going.

Some years ago, I was in North Carolina. I always go through the audience before I speak, looking at everyone. My eyes landed on a couple in the first row, and I had this urge to go over and ask them, "Where is your child?" You understand, intelligent people with "M.D." after their name don't behave this way. That is why I have a terrible reputation; people think I have slipped. This is a bad problem and I know that, but if I listened to my intellectual quadrant all the time I could never do this work.

During the first break, I went to them and said, "This may be strange to ask, but where is your child?" They answered, "We debated whether or not to bring him, but he had chemotherapy this morning." I said, "I really think he should be here." The father left and got him. The child listened a while, and then he took the paper and crayons and drew a picture. During the lunch break I sat on the steps, and he came to me and said, "Dr. Ross, here is the picture." The mother, on the verge of tears, said, "Our biggest fear was just confirmed. We were told that Dougie has maybe three months to live." I looked at the picture, and I said, "Oh no, that is totally out of the question. Maybe three years, but not three months."

After the lecture was over, I went to Dougie and told him that I couldn't make house calls in North Carolina. I said, "It's too far and costs a lot of money, but if you ever, ever need me just write and be sure to address the envelope yourself. I get thousands of letters, but the letters from children are my top priority, and if you address it I'll know it's from you." I waited and waited and the silly intellectual quadrant took over, and I started worrying that I had given the parents false hope. Then I thought, "Isn't that stupid? Whenever you let the intellectual quadrant get in the way, you are proven wrong." So I let go of the anxiety, and two days later I got a letter.

Dear Dr. Ross,

I have just two more questions.
What is life and what is death?
And why do little children have to die?

Love, Dougie

I was so touched by the beauty of its simplicity and straightforwardness. I took paper and folded it like a book. I took my daughter's felt-tipped markers, and I printed so he could read it and choose to share it or not share it with his parents. I wrote in rainbow colors because it was for a child, and then I began to illustrate it. When it was written and illustrated, I liked it, and I didn't want to give it away. I thought to myself, "It's okay. You can keep it," rationalizing that I work with many dying children. The minute you start rationalizing, you know that it's not okay. At the end of life, as you survey your life, it is not just your deeds, but also your words and your thoughts that make up the totality of your life. If you strive to always make the highest choice, you will never go wrong. I already knew that the best choice was not to keep it. So I gave myself a big kick in the pants, walked to the post office, and mailed this letter off.

Months later, I got a phone call from Dougie. "It's my birthday, and you were the only one who thought I would have another birthday. I wanted to give you something for my birthday, and I couldn't think what to give you. So I decided to send the letter back. I mailed it today."

This gift was not without conditions. There was an unspoken expectation that the card be published to help other dying children. Because I picked the higher choice at the time, this letter has now reached ten thousand dying children. This is what I tried to tell you at the beginning: If you give something of yourself without claim, it comes back ten thousand times. I mean that literally—it comes back ten thousand times. Not always through the same source, but it does come back. You may ask and not get what you think you want, but you do get what you need.

The best example I have of this is some years back when I was in San Francisco. I was really tired, and I just wanted to get home to my garden. I just needed to take care of *me*. Just as my plane was about to start boarding, this woman came and grabbed my blouse and said, "Dr. Ross?" And I so badly wanted to say, "No, I am Mary Smith." I've signed three hundred books. I've lectured to three thousand people.

One time I was at Kennedy airport, and I went to the toilet, and the moment I sat down a hand came under the door with a book, and a voice said, "Dr. Ross, would you mind?" That's no joke. That is how I live. I literally cannot pee in peace anymore. Do you understand when you live such a life that you really do just want to be Mary Smith, and you don't know why Mary Smith doesn't want to be Mary Smith? That's how I felt at that moment. I looked at this woman, and I knew that she knew that I didn't want to be me. And she said very quickly, "Dr. Ross, we just lost our nine-year-old son to cancer. Two weeks ago, after we buried him, we found out that our eleven-year-old daughter is full of cancer. We can't go through it anymore. We can't even go into her bedroom and look at her. We can't talk to her. We resent her. We can't take anymore. We need help." All I could think was "Oh God, if only I could have one hour with this couple." The second I had that thought, over the loud speaker came the announcement that Flight 83 would be delayed by one hour.

That is how your life is when you get in harmony with the four quadrants of your self. You don't have to go to church—excuse me, pastors! You don't have to be religious. We are all the same. It doesn't matter what religion, creed, what color, what income. We are all the same. We all have to go back to the same source and learn the same lessons. If you live your life this way, it will be absolutely beautiful, and you will find the strength and the energy. I am not exaggerating. You will have the strength to work seventeen-, eighteen-hour days, seven days a week, and you will never, ever get burned out. My schedule is totally inhuman, but whenever I need the strength and the energy I get absolutely and completely just what I need.

We all have repressed Hitlers inside. The greatest repressed Hitler in me was identified when I was in Maui. As much as I hate the man who showed it to me, I am forever grateful to him. Without giving you the details, somebody in Maui pushed my buttons. I was shocked because I go around teaching about unconditional love, but after a few days I was ready to put this man through the meat grinder. All week I wouldn't look at him out of fear that I would literally kill him. By the time the week ended, I was drained—totally depleted.

My next stop was Chicago where I would be spending Easter with my children, but one of my friends was meeting me in California where I changed planes. And my friend and I share a vow: We have to do our work free of charge and help when we can. And anytime you get in touch with your own unfinished business, you go home and do something about it because you can't go around preaching about it and not practice it.

So I knew she was going to ask me, and I just wanted everything to be sweet and nice with my grandchildren. And she said, "Elisabeth, how was the workshop?" And I said, "Fine." And she said, "How was the workshop?" And I said, "FINE." And she said, "How was the workshop?" And I said, "God damn it, it was fine!" And she said, "Would you like to tell me about it?" And I said, "No!" Because I wanted to get home and have things nice. Then she did the absolute worst thing that can be done to a human being when the human is feeling ugly: she was sweet. She put her hand on my head in that sweet way and said, "Tell me all about Easter bunnies." And I totally exploded. I made this big speech. "I am a psychiatrist. I am fifty years old. Don't you talk to me about Easter bunnies. I don't believe in Easter bunnies anymore. If you want to talk to your clients about Easter bunnies go ahead, but don't talk to me, a physician, about them."

Then I broke down. I emptied an ocean of tears, like I have never cried. I cried for eight hours. I regressed to a five-and-a-half-year-old child. The floodgates opened, and all of my repressed memories came up. I told her how my one sister was forever on my mother's lap and my other sister was forever on my father's lap. How if my parents really loved me they would have noticed. How I rejected them and decided to get my own hugs, stand on my own two feet. So I started to raise bunnies. And if I needed a hug, I would hold them tight. I would cry on their fur. I would tell them about the pain, the anguish, and the unfairness of the world. They would listen to me because I was the one who fed them.

My father, however, was a thrifty Swiss. Every six months or so he would get the taste for a rabbit roast and say, "Elisabeth, bring one of your rabbits to the butcher."

In those days, you did not talk back to your father. No, you picked up a rabbit and you walked the half mile down the road and you delivered it to the butcher. I was heartbroken, but I never shed a tear. Part of my arrogance was that they didn't deserve to know my pain. They didn't deserve to know how much they hurt me because it would have made me more vulnerable. The butcher always came out with a paper bag with the raw meat inside, and I would walk the half mile up the mountain and deliver it to my mother's kitchen. Then I would have to sit at the table and watch my family eat my beloved rabbit. Never shed a tear. Every time it was repeated I grew more repressed and less able to share my emotions.

When I was six and a half, I only had Blackie left. Blackie was my most beloved, so chubby and gorgeous, with such shiny fur. He was my whole love. Then the day came when my father said that I had to bring Blackie. I tried to let Blackie run away, but he loved me so much he wouldn't leave. So I took Blackie to the butcher—this brutish three-hundred-pound man with red hair and a red face. When he brought the paper bag back he said, "It is a darn shame you had to bring this rabbit. In a day or two she would have had little bunnies." You understand, I didn't even know it was a "she" bunny. But I was totally, totally devastated. I walked home like a zombie. I delivered the bag to my mother's kitchen. I sat at the dining room table like a stone. Never shed a tear. I didn't understand it then, but I can understand it now. Every time I see thrifty men, I put that lid on tighter and tighter and tighter, and it took that man in Maui to finally pop the lid. Do you understand? As much as I hate that man, I bless him.

I hope you understand what I am trying to tell you. We all have a black bunny locked up inside—you, me, all those people locked up in jail. It is my greatest hope that we can begin to help not only those in prison, but those who care for those in prison, and those of you who have compassion and understanding, to help prevent at least our next generation from going through such nightmares.

I often get asked about how to deal with children who are acting out because they have a black bunny or a repressed Hitler inside. Start a screaming room: a safe, preferably soundproof place. Give the child a three-dollar piece of vulcanized rubber hose and a mattress, and let them externalize the unfairness and rage they have bottled up. Then they will never become Hitlers in real life.

You have to help children externalize their hate and their rage without hurting living things. It's as simple as that. In the old days women would beat their carpets. Now we have vacuum cleaners. Men used to chop wood and curse. We don't do those things anymore, so we have to create places where it is okay to externalize these emotions.

I also recommend these rooms for parents who have lost children, especially directly after hearing the news. Once the physician has informed the family, they can be taken to a screaming room. We have done this in several hospitals and have staffed the screaming room with members of Compassionate Friends, people who have not been trained by books and theories, but by life. They were in the parents' place themselves two years ago, three years ago, five years ago. They come back and say, "I have recuperated and I want to do something for other people." Those people come in and they are the only people (with very few exceptions) that practice unconditional love to the grieving parents, because they remember that it was what they needed.

Some parents are numb and have to be allowed to be so. Some become very businesslike and want to call everyone. Some need to scream and curse everything and everyone, including God. No one should tell them not to do that; God is strong enough to take it. Who are you to come to God's defense? They must be allowed to externalize their feelings without being judged. If they are allowed to get it out, you will never have the tragedies that we hear about in our workshops.

A month later, the people who staff the screaming room call the families and ask, "Do you feel like talking?" Because when you are just informed of a murder or a suicide or an accidental death or a coronary or whatever, you are sometimes in a state of shock or numbness. You don't really think. After all of the relatives have gone home and the funeral is over and the neighbors have stopped cooking and the pastor has stopped visiting, it's like a defrosting. It's like it suddenly begins to hit you. "Oh my God, it really is true. He is never going to come home again." That is when all the questions come up. So they call, and they always ask the same questions: Was he alive when he was found? Was somebody with him? Did somebody hold his hand? You answer their questions, and they thank you. Done this way, grief resolution is much, much faster.

Our research in life after death shows that no human being can die alone. So do not sit on your guilt that you were not with your loved ones at the moment of death, because all of that is irrelevant. The moment you die, you leave your physical body. Anybody you need to be with, you can be with even if they are ten thousand miles away. If I were to die here and think of my sister in Switzerland, I would be there in the split second it takes to think of my sister. No one can die alone.

Say you are in an accident and you shed your physical body. You look down at the scene. You are aware of the accident. You are aware of the blowtorch they are using to extricate your body. You have no pain, no panic, no fear, no anxiety, no grief, and no negative feelings. All you have is a sense of "Wow! A lot of people are working on my body." Then you realize that you are aware of the resuscitation team, but the resuscitation team is not aware of you.

You begin to become aware not only that you are whole again, but also that you can be anywhere you want to be. That is why dying children send their mommies and daddies home before they die. Because mommies and daddies often lean over the side rail and implicitly or explicitly say, "Honey, don't die on me. I can't live without you." They make the child feel guilty for dying, which makes it very hard to let go. Since the children already know that they can be with Mommy and

Daddy anyway, they return to their bodies and say, "Why don't you go home? Take a shower and rest. I am really all right." And they are all right. Not the way we want them to be all right, but they are all right. Then the phone call comes. "I'm sorry. Suzy died." The parents pull their hair out, "Why didn't we stay another half hour?" Little do they know that Suzy did this in order to let go, knowing that she is going to be with them forever anyway.

You are met by those who preceded you in death—mother, father, grandmother, grandfather. You see first those who you loved the most. A man once said to me, "I have a big problem. My God! I had eight wives." I hope you understand that problems like this are earthly problems. On the "other side" such problems don't exist. The only thing that counts is love. My youngest patient was a two-year-old boy from a Catholic family who shared with his mother that he had been in the most beautiful place. He did not want to come back because he was with Jesus and Mary. Mary kept telling him that the time was not right, that he had to go back. He tried to ignore her, which is very typical of any two-year-old. When Mary realized that he would not listen to her, she took him gently by the wrist and said, "Peter, you must go back. You have to save your mommy." Peter later said, "You know, Mommy, when she told me that, I ran all the way home." You understand, a Protestant child would not see Mary, and a non-Christian would not see Jesus. You always see first whoever you loved the most.

A woman was hit by a drunk driver. A man stopped and asked if he could help, and she said, "No, there is nothing you can do for me." Then she said, "On second thought, maybe one day you will go to the reservation. If you do, do me a favor. Find my mother and give her a message. Tell her that I was okay. That I was not only okay but very happy because I am already with my dad." She died in the arms of this total stranger. The man was so moved that he drove seven hundred miles out of his way to the Native American reservation. He found the mother who told him that her husband had died of an unexpected coronary an hour before the car accident in which the daughter was killed. This case gave me the idea to begin this research.

From then on, I spent a lot of time in hospital intensive care units. I always picked the youngest children who had not been told who else was killed at the scene of the accident, how many parents, aunts, uncles, grandparents, brothers, or sisters had been killed. Just before these children died, they had a glimpse and were no longer afraid. When you work with people in this condition, you can tell when this takes place. There is a peace and serenity about them.

All I ever say to them is "Is there anything that you can share with me?" A young boy once said, "Everything is okay now. My mommy and Peter are waiting for me." I knew that his mother had died in the accident, but his brother Peter had not. Peter was badly burned and sent to another hospital. In all the years I have done research in death and dying and life after death, I have never seen a child in this situation make a mistake, so I simply accept that reality. As I was walking out past the nurses' station, the telephone call came. "Dr. Ross, I just wanted to tell you that Peter died ten minutes ago from his burns." I naturally say, "Yes, I know," and they think I'm a kook. Do you understand what I am trying to say to you? Dying is not a nightmare—what we make for one another right here in this life is the nightmare.

There's a beautiful poem by a woman whose fiancé went to Vietnam, which I will paraphrase for you—"Honey, do you remember when I wanted to go to the beach, and you said, 'No, it's going to rain all day'? And I insisted, 'We are going to the beach.' And you finally came along and it rained all day. And I thought you were really going to let me have it, but you didn't. Do you remember when I insisted that we go to that dance but you really didn't want to go? And I said, 'We are going to that dance.' And you came, but I forgot to tell you that it was formal and you came in blue jeans. And I thought you were going to kill me. But you didn't. Do you remember when I desperately tried to make you jealous by going out with this other guy that you couldn't stand? And I thought you were going to leave me, but you didn't. I wanted to tell you all this when you came back from Vietnam, but you didn't."

Richard Allen had the same insight after the death of his father with whom he never really communicated. The last few lines of his poem:

> When you love, give it everything you've got.
> And when you have reached your limit, give it more,
> and forget the pain of it.
> Because as you face your death
> it is only the love that you have given and received
> which will count,
> and all the rest:
> the accomplishments, the struggle, the fights
> will be forgotten in your reflection.
> And if you have loved well
> then it will all have been worth it.
> And the joy of it will last you until the end.
> But if you have not,
> death will always come too soon
> and be too terrible to face.

Creating a Dharma Vision 5

Anyen Rinpoche

Deepening Our Commitment to Dharma Practice

It seems timely and useful now, regardless of our age, to focus on our personal progress since taking up the Buddhist path. How have we changed? How have we worked with obstacles that have arisen along the way? Have we slipped back into any unwholesome habitual patterns and not even noticed? What kind of faith do we find in our hearts right now? What is our current commitment to practice? Where do we want to be as Dharma practitioners at the time of our death?

These are not just rhetorical questions. Please ask them to yourself, right now. Take an honest look inside and recognize what you need to do to fulfill your spiritual aspirations in whatever time you have left. All of these questions together are what is meant by the question "What is your Dharma Vision?" What kind of practitioner are you *truly* willing to become so that the moment of death fulfills the aspirations you have for enlightenment—or at the very least to take a rebirth that allows you to continue your practice and be in the presence of authentic teachers again?

Just as all of us make great effort to maintain our everyday lives, we should make similarly great effort in our preparations for death. If we are living and practicing the essence of the Dharma teachings, there should be no difference between our spiritual practices while we are living and those that we engage in at the time of death. One practice that we all share on the path, no matter what other teachings we have received or practices we have committed to, is training in mindfulness to ensure that in our last moments we will be able to make good use of our death.

We all seek to be the best human beings we can be. And regardless of our beliefs, death will come to all of us. Everyone can benefit from preparing for death as a spiritual practice. Additionally, if we learn how to support a loved one while they are dying, we will be giving them a great gift by helping them fulfill their own spiritual aspirations.

The Need for a Dharma Vision

Many of us on the Buddhist path have heard from our teachers that "the path is the goal" and that we should cut through any attachments to results. This is most true specifically on the path of meditation; we should not have hope for any particular experiences or signs of realization in our meditation. Hungering for such experiences will only bring us obstacles. Nevertheless, without earnest self-reflection and a vision for ourselves as practitioners, we will not really know how to take up the path.

We must be careful about having only the *appearance* of a Dharma practitioner. Some students who have received many teachings tell me they are "on and off" practitioners; they "sort of" practice and have little experience. Sometimes they are very passionate about one practice for a short period of time. They may burn like fire, but then something or other happens and they stop practicing. They lack certainty about what is the perfectly pure path. We need to abandon this habit of being an "on and off" practitioner. If we let our energy get too high, we can expect a counterbalancing low to follow when we lose our enthusiasm. Thus, in terms of Dharma practice, having a tempered passion is a more useful quality.

Because it is so easy to deceive ourselves about our practice, it is very important to have a relationship with a spiritual friend, a lama, who will help cut through any self-deception. But we must do our part to be prepared for and to nurture such a relationship; we must be diligent in our practice and have a realistic idea of our spiritual goals. Self-reflection can bring a new level of trust and mutual respect to an established relationship with a teacher by demonstrating that we are suitable spiritual "vessels," worthy of receiving profound lineage teachings. We can transform our outer trust in the Three Jewels—in the Buddha, in the teachings, and in the community of noble practitioners—into authentic confidence that develops unshakable faith in the Buddhist path to enlightenment.

I consider the Dharma Vision, what we might call our spiritual aspirations, to be an evolving meditation on living and dying. It makes no difference what stage of life we are in. As practitioners, we need a guide for living as well as for dying that we can skillfully rely on during our lives as well as at the moment of death.

It's also important to include others in our Dharma Vision. Many of us, wishing to increase our expressions of loving-kindness and compassion, also want to help friends, loved ones, pets, and strangers alike die with the same opportunities for a "good death" that we wish for ourselves. If we do have the wish to help others through the dying process, we must first train ourselves to understand how our own lives move toward death. We must gain knowledge and wisdom about the process of dying that will enable us to use one of the most important moments of this incarnation wisely. Then we can make a serious commitment to becoming practitioners who take responsibility for accomplishing the vision of helping ourselves and others to die well.

At the end of this chapter is a special section with contemplations and guided meditations to help you develop and clarify your Dharma Vision.

The Dharma Will, Entrusted Dharma Friends, and the Dharma Box

When we understand the importance of the dying process and the potential we have for liberation during and after our death, it will be easy to see how essential it is to prepare properly for death. I would like to plant seeds here first for the ideas of a Dharma Will and of what I call entrusted Dharma friends.

I encourage students to form core groups of entrusted Dharma friends who agree to help each other through the dying process according to the wishes written down in each person's Dharma Will. The Dharma Will allows us to record our spiritual directives, so family and friends will know the kind of death we wish to experience and how it can be accomplished. Once each person has written a Dharma Will, he or she can share it within the core group as part of training in recognizing the signs of death, mastering the important practices, and learning how to skillfully help someone through the dying process.

Entire sanghas, or spiritual communities, can also pledge to help entrusted Dharma friends within their community fulfill their commitments. Each core group will need others from the spiritual community to assume some of the tasks involved in supporting the dying person's wishes, such as informing the sangha about appropriate prayers and rituals, practicing together, and helping with funeral arrangements. This will be a wonderful way to strengthen our spiritual relationships and gain confidence in using the dying process for spiritual practice.

I also advocate creating a "Dharma Box," an actual box that will contain everything we and our entrusted Dharma friends will need to help us through the dying process. The Dharma Box will include copies of our Dharma Will and legal papers, ritual items, Dharma practice texts, and instructions for family and friends. Once the Dharma Box is complete, we can return to our Dharma Vision and engage fully in the practices we have committed to through the creation of that vision, with the assurance that we have put everything in place for the time of death.

Creating Your Dharma Vision through Contemplation

There are many traditional meditations on death and impermanence. We can think about how the seasons change and how the elements of the world around us transform; we can look at how our bodies have changed from the time we were born until now; we can contemplate how our minds are constantly transforming. Reflecting on impermanence is the best way to prepare ourselves for the moment of death; please take some time to reflect on the contemplations below.

In the next few pages, I will suggest some specific questions for students to contemplate. It would be best to set aside a personal retreat day or weekend without interruptions for these practices, or to do this with your entrusted Dharma friends in a group retreat. You may want a journal to write down insights and ideas that arise as you do these practices. Some students have also found journaling helpful in tracking their progress in meditation and conduct over a period of a month or so, and they use that as a basis for further reflection. You should decide what tools will help you the most in making this assessment of your Dharma practice.

Again, I encourage you to take an honest look at yourself as a Buddhist practitioner on the path. Sit quietly and cultivate a proper motivation. Generate *bodhichitta*—the wish to become enlightened in order to help others attain enlightenment—for all sentient beings. I suggest you read one of the contemplations below to yourself a few times over. Take time to consider it fully, keeping your mind focused but open to all ideas that arise. When you feel ready, rest in meditation free of reference points for as long as you can. When you finish your meditation, if you like, take time to write about your insights and experiences. Then continue with the next contemplation in the same way.

When you've thoroughly explored each of the contemplations below, you can begin to incorporate what you have learned about yourself as a practitioner into your Dharma Vision. Even if you have been practicing for a long time, you may be surprised at what you find lacking in your practice when you have taken an honest look. Many of my students find great inspiration in this process to increase their diligence and focus on areas needing attention. Don't forget to practice compassion for yourself. Appreciate the past efforts you have already made and include the efforts you are willing to make to become the excellent practitioner you have envisioned.

One of the biggest obstacles we might find we have as practitioners is that we lack a sense of urgency about the need to practice. This is caused by our strong experience of self-attachment. Self-attachment is expressed in many different ways. For example, we might think, "Let me just enjoy my life right now; let me enjoy this particular moment." We put off practice for a later time, which we fail to realize may never come. The best time to practice, the best time to prepare for the reality of death, and the best time to clarify our own Dharma Visions is the present. Don't waste a moment.

Having a sense of urgency about practice could cause us to overestimate ourselves, however, or to want to skip over the hard work of developing a solid and stable base of daily practice. As you create your Dharma Vision, make an effort to balance idealism with realism. We may all wish to be great yogis like Milarepa or Longchenpa, but our capacity is more likely to be one of an ordinary practitioner. We should reflect realistically on where we are now in our practice and what kind of practitioner we wish to become. We must be honest about our capacity so that our goal will not be beyond our reach. As I have stated above, we must also continually be mindful of life's impermanence and the reality of impending death. We may not have all the time we think we will have to practice.

We can aspire to such goals as receiving profound instructions from authentic teachers of all lineages and gaining experience and certainty in their meaning and in the primordially pure view of Dzogchen. We can always aspire to increase our bodhichitta and can do so by daily employing such practices as *tonglen*, in which we take in the suffering of others and send out positive wishes for healing and happiness in exchange. We all should wish to become proficient at practicing *phowa*, or transference of consciousness, for ourselves so that we may use it effectively at the time of our deaths, to die without regrets and with altruistic motivation for our next life. We may wish to become a practitioner who can sit with confidence with people who are dying and support them during the dying process. We may think about how we may help our teachers accomplish their Dharma activities and where we can contribute our talents.

Regardless of how we regard our talent for writing, we can all compose an aspiration prayer for the time of our death and include it at the end of the Dharma Vision. We can read this aspiration prayer before sleep each night so its meaning fully enters our hearts. Then, as we are dying, an entrusted Dharma friend can read this to us to remind us of what we are trying to accomplish and of our bodhichitta. A copy of this prayer can be kept in our Dharma Box and buried or burned with us after we die.

Ideas to Contemplate

CONTEMPLATE IMPERMANENCE FROM THE OUTER POINT OF VIEW

▷ Reflect on how your outer environment has changed during the past year. Recall how the seasons changed: how the plants, flowers, and trees transformed over time; how the daylight increased and decreased. Think about it both in your own personal living environment and throughout the globe as well. Think about the natural catastrophes that occurred around the world. Reflect on all the births and deaths of people, animals, and insects. Allow the enormity of these changes to reach you on a deep level until you feel with certainty that not even one thing remained the same.

CONTEMPLATE IMPERMANENCE FROM THE INNER POINT OF VIEW

▷ Imagine yourself as a small baby. See the physical changes you have gone through until now. Sometimes looking at photos of yourself from childhood to the present can be a poignant way to examine your own physical impermanence. Look at the transformation that has occurred in you physically. Then think about your physical being from last year until now, from last month until now, from yesterday until today. See that your body is changing even from moment to moment.

CONTEMPLATE IMPERMANENCE FROM THE SECRET POINT OF VIEW

▷ Reflect on the wild nature of your own mind. Remember yourself as a child and how your intelligence developed over time. Look at how your mind changes moment by moment as it fills with entertaining distractions or follows after different sensory experiences. Contemplate how you are constantly transforming mentally and how the mind is also impermanent.

CONTEMPLATE YOUR SPIRITUAL PRACTICE

▷ Reflect on your daily practice. Are you practicing regularly and for as long as you would like? Are you able to incorporate all the practices you wish to master into your daily practice?

Reflect deeply on what type of practitioner you really want to be. What are the obstacles that stand in your way? Think about any tendencies you have that prevent you from practicing in this way. What is the main cause? Identify the things that cause you to put off practicing.

CONTEMPLATE THE IMPERMANENCE OF THINGS TO WHICH YOU ARE ATTACHED

▷ If you are attached to material objects in the world around you, reflect on their changing nature. If you are attached to a person, reflect on him or her growing old and dying. Actually envision his or her physical and mental changes. If you are attached to your own life, as we all are, go through your body from the ends of the hair on your head to the tips of your toes and try to find anything that is lasting or permanent in your body. Do a very thorough examination, looking from outside to inside to see if you can find anything that is unchanging. Do this until you are confident that you, too, are actually going to die, and that you cannot hold on to this life forever.

CONTEMPLATE THE SIX PARAMITAS, OR TRANSCENDENT ACTIONS, STARTING WITH THIS PAST MONTH'S PRACTICE OF GENEROSITY

▷ Look at how you practiced during the past month and how you have integrated practice into your daily life by examining how you have expressed generosity. Were you able to give love, emotional support, or material goods without attachment? Was your heart open unconditionally? If you compare this month to the previous month, was your generosity different or the same? If you compare last year to this year, have you been more generous? Less generous? The same? If you are the same, what will you do to increase your expression of generosity? If you have been less generous, reflect on why you have changed.

CONTEMPLATE THIS PAST MONTH'S SPIRITUAL PRACTICE IN TERMS OF THE REMAINING PARAMITAS

▷ In the same way, examine your progress in virtue and morality; patience and tolerance; diligence and enthusiastic effort; meditative concentration; and wisdom. Take time to look at each quality and how you express it in your daily life. If you find yourself lacking in the expression of these enlightened qualities, make a plan to work on them. For example, make an effort to stay mindful of one quality over the next month and look for ways to enhance it. You will find many opportunities. Over time you can become habituated to remaining mindful and increasing the practice of each quality. You will find your daily practice improving greatly.

CONTEMPLATE THIS PAST MONTH'S SPIRITUAL PRACTICE IN TERMS OF ANGER

▷ It is very important to similarly contemplate your recent expressions of anger and resentment. These are the hardest to purify. Compare your expressions of anger and resentment in the past to how you feel currently. As a general trend, is it becoming easier to let go of them and generate compassion? If not, how will you work on this? Again, focus on anger or resentment by remaining mindful as these emotions arise. Work with any methods you have been given to cut through afflictive emotions. If this is difficult for you, ask your spiritual friend for advice.

CONTEMPLATE THIS PAST MONTH'S SPIRITUAL PRACTICE IN TERMS OF THE VIEW

▹ If you have received instructions from your lama on abiding in the view, or the nature of mind, assess your progress during the past month. Were you able to remember to abide in the view one hundred times a day? Twenty-one times a day? Three times? Have you increased the number of times you remembered to practice? Has it become easier? If not, how will you improve your practice?

CONTEMPLATE THE IMPORTANCE OF MASTERING THE MIND

▹ Your mind must deal with every experience. Think about how attaining mastery over the mind will enable you to lose any fear of death. Come to the certainty that you must master your mind in order to die with confidence.

CONTEMPLATE THE DEATH OF A PET OR ANIMAL YOU LOVE

▹ Imagine that an animal you love very much is ill and close to dying. Or, considering what is happening in our world today, think that the last of an entire species you love is about to die. Recognize that animals have no way to take care of themselves spiritually or mentally in this situation. It is not that they do not want to; they are simply incapable of doing so. With compassion for their suffering, also reflect on your good fortune in being born as a human being who can take care of yourself emotionally and spiritually at the time of death.

CONTEMPLATE THE DEATH OF A PERSON YOU LOVE

▹ You may have already experienced the death of someone to whom you were very close. Perhaps they did not have all the spiritual support they needed to die without fear or regret. If so, recall the experience of their death and again reflect on the good fortune that you are able to prepare well for your own death. If you have not had someone close to you die, imagine the death of someone you love and reflect deeply on your wish that they will experience no suffering and have all the support they need to die mindfully.

CONTEMPLATE THE CAUSES AND CONDITIONS THAT LED TO YOUR BIRTH AND WILL LEAD TO YOUR DEATH

▷ Recognize the long chain of positive and negative actions that brings you to this very moment. Search for a deep understanding of karma, causes and conditions, and how you can affect your spiritual path with mindful actions from now until death. Then consider the type of practitioner you wish to be at your death and what kind of spiritual support you will want from others. Take time to imagine yourself in the dying process. Do you have the confidence to die well? Are you ready?

Also, reflect on the idea that you may die suddenly, or during an accident. How can you be spiritually prepared for that experience?

CONTEMPLATE DIFFICULTIES WITH YOUR DEATH

▷ As you imagine yourself dying, do any obstacles arise in your mind that would prevent you from having the kind of death you wish? What are they and what can you do to remove them?

CONTEMPLATE YOUR IDEAL DEATH

▷ What will your mind be like? What qualities will you have developed? What practice will be most important for you to do or hear at that time? Who do you want to be there to help you stay focused on your practice as you are dying?

CONTEMPLATE YOUR LEVEL OF PRACTICE

▷ What changes do you need to make in your daily practice to best ensure you become the type of practitioner you want to be?

CONTEMPLATE YOUR RELATIONSHIP WITH A SPIRITUAL FRIEND

▷ If you have had the good fortune to meet and make a strong connection to a lama or spiritual teacher, reflect on this relationship and what it is like now. Have you developed the kind of relationship you envision? If not, what can you do to develop this relationship further?

Revising Your Dharma Vision

The Dharma Vision is a living and evolving meditation. We are always changing and growing in our understanding. I recommend that each year, perhaps at the new year or on your birthday, you commit to reviewing your vision as a Dharma practitioner, assessing your progress, and seeing if there is anything new you want to add. You may want to again return to the contemplations above. If you have done any of this work in a group retreat, it would be fruitful for everyone to meet again to review and share both your progress and your obstacles. Support each other with kindness and appreciate the efforts everyone has made. Your sangha and entrusted Dharma friends are most precious!

Lucky

Tony Hoagland

If you are lucky in this life,
you will get to help your enemy
the way I got to help my mother
when she was weakened past the point of saying no.

Into the big enamel tub
half-filled with water
which I had made just right,
I lowered the childish skeleton
she had become.

Her eyelids fluttered as I soaped and rinsed
her belly and her chest,
the sorry ruin of her flanks
and the frayed gray cloud
between her legs.

Some nights, sitting by her bed
book open in my lap
while I listened to the air
move thickly in and out of her dark lungs,
my mind filled up with praise
as lush as music,

amazed at the symmetry and luck
that would offer me the chance to pay
my heavy debt of punishment and love
with love and punishment.

And once I held her dripping wet
in the uncomfortable air
between the wheelchair and the tub,
until she begged me like a child

to stop,
an act of cruelty which we both understood
was the ancient irresistible rejoicing
of power over weakness.

If you are lucky in this life,
you will get to raise the spoon
of pristine, frosty ice cream
to the trusting creature mouth
of your old enemy

because the tastebuds at least are not broken
because there is a bond between you
and sweet is sweet in any language.

Medicine

Tony Hoagland

The black hair of my Chinese doctor
gleams like combed ink
as he leans over his desk,
with quick pen strokes writing my prescription
in the lingo of the *I Ching,*
the page looks like a street
lined with sampans and pagodas,
rickshaws gliding through the palace gates
bearing Szechuan takeout to the king.

Daydreaming comes easy to the ill:
slowed down to the speed of waiting rooms,
you learn to hang suspended in the wallpaper,
to drift among the magazines and plants,
feeling a strange love
for the time that might be killing you.

Two years ago, I was so infatuated
with my lady doctor, Linda,
I wanted to get better just to please her,
and yet to go on getting worse,
to keep her leaning toward me,
with her sea green eyes and stethoscope, asking
Does that hurt?

Does it hurt? Yes, it hurts
so sweet. It hurts exquisitely.

It hurts real good. I feel as if I read it
in some Bible for the ill,
that suffering itself is medicine
and to endure enough will cure you
of anything.

So I want more injury
and repair, an ulcer
and a migraine, please.
I want to suffer like my mother,

who said once, following a shot
—her face joyful as the needle entered—
that she felt a train had been injected
straight into her vein. Day after day,
to see her sinking
through the layers of our care

was to learn something delicious
about weakness:
as if she had discovered
the train was bound somewhere;
as if the conductor
had told everyone on board
they never had to bear the weight
of being strong again.

Meeting the Divine Messengers 6

Bhikkhu Bodhi

The traditional legend of the Buddha's life tells us that throughout his youth and early manhood Prince Siddhattha, the Bodhisatta, lived completely unaware of the most elementary facts concerning human mortality. His father, anxious to protect his sensitive son from exposure to suffering, kept him an unwitting captive of ignorance. Incarcerated in the splendor of his palace, amply supplied with sensual pleasures, and surrounded by merry friends, the prince did not entertain even the faintest suspicion that life could offer anything other than an endless succession of amusements and festivities. It was only on that fateful day in his twenty-ninth year, when curiosity led him out beyond the palace walls, that he encountered the four "divine messengers" that were to change his destiny. The first three were the old man, the sick man, and the corpse, which taught him the shocking truths of old age, illness, and death; the fourth was a wandering ascetic, who revealed to him the existence of a path whereby all suffering can be fully overcome.

This charming story, which has nurtured the faith of Buddhists through the centuries, enshrines at its heart a profound psychological truth. In the language of myth it speaks to us, not merely of events that may have taken place centuries ago, but of a process of awakening through which each of us must pass if the Dhamma is to come to life within ourselves. Beneath the symbolic veneer of the ancient legend we can see that Prince Siddhattha's youthful stay in the palace was not so different from the way in which most of us today pass our entire lives—often, sadly, until it is too late to strike out in a new direction.

Our homes may not be royal palaces, and the wealth at our disposal may not approach anywhere near that of a North Indian rajah, but we share with the young Prince Siddhattha a blissful (and often willful) oblivion to stark realities that are constantly thrusting themselves on our attention. If the teachings are to be more than the bland, humdrum background of a comfortable life, if they are to become the inspiring, sometimes grating, voice that steers us on to the great path of awakening, we ourselves need to emulate the Bodhisatta in his process of maturation. Joining him on his journey outside the palace walls—the walls of our own self-assuring preconceptions—we must see for ourselves the divine messengers we so often miss because our eyes are fixed on "more important things," i.e., on our mundane preoccupations and goals.

The Buddha says that there are few who are stirred by things that are truly stirring, compared to those, far more numerous, who are not so stirred. The spurs to awakening press in on us from all sides, yet too often, instead of acknowledging them, we respond simply by putting on another layer of clothes to protect ourselves from their sting. This statement is not disproved even by the recent deluge of discussion and literature on aging, life-threatening illnesses, and alternative approaches to death and dying. Open and honest awareness is still not sufficient for the divine messengers to get their message across. To convey their message, the message that can goad us on to the path to liberation, something more is needed. We must confront aging, illness, and death not simply as inescapable realities with which we must somehow cope at the practical level but as envoys from the beyond, from the far shore, disclosing new dimensions of meaning.

This disclosure takes place at two levels. First, to become divine messengers, the facts of aging, illness, and death must jolt us into an awareness of the fragile, precarious nature of our normal day-to-day lives. The first three messengers must impress upon our minds the radical deficiency that runs through all our worldly concerns, extending to conditioned existence in its totality. Thereby they become windows opening upon the first noble truth, the noble truth of suffering, which the Buddha says comprises not only birth, aging, illness, and death, not only sorrow, grief, pain, and misery, but all the physical and mental factors that make up our being-in-the-world. The homeless ascetic must become more than a quaint object of curiosity; he should serve us as a reminder that the way to liberation cuts through the austere landscape of renunciation and inner self-mastery. Clad in his ochre robes, this sedate and dignified figure serves as a pointer to the fourth noble truth, the truth of the path, and its culmination, the truth of suffering's cessation.

When we meet the divine messengers at this level, they become catalysts that can induce in us a profound internal transformation. We realize that because we are frail and inescapably mortal we must make drastic changes in our existential priorities and personal values. Instead of letting our lives be consumed by transient trivia, by things that are here today and gone tomorrow, we must give weight to "what really counts," to aims and actions that will exert a lasting influence upon our long-range destinies and our ultimate aim as we meander through the cycle of repeated birth and death.

Before such a revaluation takes place, we generally live in a condition that the Buddha describes by the term *pamāda*: negligence or heedlessness. Imagining ourselves immortal, and the world our personal playground, we devote our energies to such "worldy dharmas" as the accumulation of wealth, the enjoyment of sensual pleasures, the achievement of status, the quest for fame and renown. The remedy for heedlessness is the very same quality that was aroused in the Bodhisatta when he met the divine messengers in the streets of Kapilavatthu. This quality, called in Pali *samvega*, is a "sense of urgency," an inner commotion or shock that does not allow us to rest content with our habitual adjustment to the world. Instead it drives us on to embark on our own journey into homelessness, whether actual or metaphoric. As Prince Siddhattha did after meeting the homeless mendicant, we must leave behind our cozy palaces and plunge into unfamiliar jungles, to work out with diligence an authentic solution to our existential plight.

It is at this point that the second function of the divine messengers comes to prominence. For aging, sickness, and death are not only emblems of the unsatisfactory nature of mundane existence but pointers to a deeper reality that lies beyond. In the traditional legend the four divine messengers are gods in disguise. They have been sent down to Earth from the highest heaven to awaken the Bodhisatta to his momentous mission, and once they have delivered their message they resume their celestial forms. This teaches us that the final word of the Dhamma is not surrender, not an injunction to resign ourselves to the cruel fact of our human mortality, nor even to accept our finitude in a mood of joyful celebration. The inevitability of old age, sickness, and death is the preliminary message of the Dhamma, the announcement that our house is ablaze. The final message, suggested by the fourth divine messenger, is something else: an ebullient cry that there is a place of safety, an open field beyond the flames, and a clear exit sign pointing the way of escape.

If, in this process of awakening, we must meet old age, sickness, and death face to face, that is because the place of safety can be reached only by honest confrontation with the harsh truths about human existence. We cannot reach safety by pretending that the flames that engulf our home are nothing but bouquets of flowers: we must see them as they are, as real flames. When, however, we do look at the divine messengers squarely, without embarrassment or fear, we will find that their faces undergo an unexpected metamorphosis. Before our eyes, by subtle degrees, they change into another face—the face of the Buddha, with its serene smile of triumph over the army of Mara, over the demons of Desire and Death. The divine messengers point to what lies beyond the transient, to a dimension of reality where there is no more aging, no more sickness, and no more death. This is the goal and final destination of the Buddhist path—Nibbāna, the Unaging, the Illness-free, the Deathless. It is to direct us there that the divine messengers have appeared in our midst, and their message is the good news that this goal is available to us.

7 The Healing Encounter: Meeting One Another in the Space Between

Judy Lief

We are all healed. We start out healed: we are fundamentally healed, and we have never been un-healed.

Basic healthiness is our fundamental nature. The word *heal* is not just connected to getting over a disease, it is connected to the word *whole*. It is about wholeness. We are whole and complete no matter what our condition or so-called state of health and illness might be. The word *heal* is also connected to the word *holy*. So it evokes the recognition of the sacred quality of this precious life: the sacredness of our bodies, our minds, and our emotions, no matter what their condition of chaos, pleasure, or pain may be.

So what does it really mean to be healed? What keeps us from being healed? I know people who have been cured of illness who are very much healed, and I know people who seem to "recover" who are very much not healed. What does it take to feel whole? What would it mean to be at ease instead of in a state of dis-ease, out of balance, out of ease? What would it mean to be fully at ease in your own skin, in your own state of mind, however it is, and your own state of health, no matter what it is?

In looking at the role of caregivers—or healers, clinicians, doctors, nurses, or whatever you want to call it—in relationship with patients there really are no doctors, and there are no patients. There really aren't! There are just humans who have certain roles to play. However, I think these roles become the reality, and the actual humans become less real. So how can we connect? How can we encounter one another from those positions, from conventional notions of what it is to be a teacher or a minister or a rabbi or a doctor or a patient? We have ideas of what such encounters are supposed to be like, what others are supposed to be like, what we are supposed to be like. And the way we talk about these things in our culture very much affects the nature of our experience. We talk about success or failure, we talk about winning or losing. We speak in terms of battles, of losing the battle against cancer or winning the battle against cancer. We have embarrassment and we have fear.

The word *encounter* is related to *contra* as in *contrary*. There is a sense of contrast, of two sides coming together from different perspectives, like a crash. So perhaps a better term, instead of the healing encounter, would be the healing space or healing inter-being. Thich Nhat Hanh's term *interbeing* points to our interconnectedness. Inter-being, being together. So if you have two people, one of them being treated, one of them being the healer, so to speak, each of them brings to the encounter their whole history, their whole religious tradition, their whole background, their whole emotional bundle—the whole enchilada. When healer and patient come into proximity, how does it change from just being in proximity to *interbeing*? How does it become a genuine encounter? And why bother? What's the point of such an encounter?

Connection matters, for this place of meeting is where the healing takes place. In my tradition, we talk a lot about "in-between" spaces. In between you and me is where healing takes place. In between past and future is where healing takes place. In that in-between, you step into raw uncomfortable space together, and that is where healing takes place. It takes place in between, the space between.

True healing—and truly being with another person—is kind of scary and vulnerable. So most of us (at least me) don't want to go there that often. Yet often we expect the other person to do so. We expect the other person to grow through the experience, and we want to watch and enjoy it from a slight distance. But how can you ask someone to go into a space that you yourself are not willing to enter?

The basic state we all share is that none of us are here that long. The world has gone on a long time without us, and it will be fine when we leave. We don't have much time. We may feel blessed in many ways of health and vigor, but this life is unpredictable—it is totally unpredictable. So how can we help ourselves be able to connect at a level that is even? Can we relate in a way that is not based on higher/lower, powerful/unpowerful, healthy/sick? Can we be in the same boat, on a level playing field with one another?

In healthcare, it's not easy because on a literal, practical, physical level you have a vertical person and a horizontal person. That is not a normal way of communicating. One person is up higher looking down at someone who is prone. Since sick people are often lying down, bedridden, right away there is a physical obstacle to operating on a level playing field.

Three Modes of Connection: Physical, Emotional, Mental

Physicality and Environment

In talking about entering together into a space that could be healing, we have three areas that we can work with, three modes of connection. The first is the physical.

It's easy to get stuck in our heads. We're trying to solve problems, we're trying to do the right thing, say the right thing, think the right thing. We think the way we'll be helpful is by having some kind of answer, some kind of pointer, something to say. And we often forget the simple physical level of connection. We forget the power of physical communication and lose track of our physicality, our bodies.

Just your simple physical entry into a room, if you are visiting someone, communicates a tremendous amount. In the first instant a person enters the room and approaches you, something is communicated. We don't often realize how much we are communicating that we are not intending to communicate. Instead of ignoring this dimension, we could make use of it by being not only more aware of what we are manifesting physically, but more intentional in what we are communicating. We do so by grounding ourselves physically, becoming more embodied, more aware of the physical presence of both ourselves and others.

Cultivating physical connectedness has to do with becoming more sophisticated about how you hold your own body, how you handle your world and the objects within it with awareness and tenderness. But it also involves being more tuned in to the effect of forms and the physical environment on healing. This is very literal. Many people spend the last days of their lives in hospital rooms within institutions that are loud, impersonal, and unpleasant. Lights shine day and night, and there are constant interruptions. They sometimes feel like places of broken glass and sharp edges. Although a hospital is a place where people go to heal, the harshness of the physical environment creates a real obstacle.

Regrouping yourself physically takes very little time. A quick touch-in before you enter the room of the person you are working with can shift the tone of the whole encounter. You could start simply, from the bottom up, from your embodiment, from your ground. Are you in your body? Are you breathing? Are you restless? Are you feeling tired or dull? Where are you in your body? Then, as you begin your encounter, you could stay with the level of physicality and embodiment as you shift your attention to the other person or persons. What is your sense of empathy with the embodied being that you are encountering, simply as a physical presence? Can you be with another simply as a person with various physical sensations, shifting like the weather?

Emotions and Energies

The second mode of connection is emotional.

It is essential to be aware of the emotional realm we share with one another. We live in a sea of emotions all the time. Sometimes these emotions are obvious and flashy, and many other times they are more like an undercurrent, gurgling beneath our consciousness in a murky way, yet coloring everything we do before we even know it.

When you enter a room, when you initiate an encounter, how receptive are you to the emotional flavor of that very moment in that very room? Are you also aware of the emotional texture within your own state of being? What emotional colors are mixing in that space of connectedness? What energies? The underpinning of emotional life to a large degree is a constant and ever-swirling pattern of hopes and fears, which feeds emotional upheavals. What hopes and fears are you carrying in with you? If you recognize or acknowledge them right off the bat, you can lessen their power.

We could look at the different emotions in terms of the good, the bad, and the ugly. In terms of positive emotions, we could speak of love, friendliness, and kindness. Those are all emotions that very much matter. We don't have to be so highfalutin as to speak of compassion—we could be simpler than that. Simple friendliness, simple kindness, goes a long way. Kindness and simplicity, simplicity and kindness.

The challenge of tuning in emotionally—to our own emotions and others—is not only to recognize what is happening, but to just be with it. Emotions are not necessarily a problem, and death does not necessarily have to be tidy. It is not as if we are being good housekeepers and we are trying to make everyone be comfortable. Attachment to comfort and emotional tidiness is something to be very much aware of. It is always good to ask: Whose comfort are we talking about here? Is it my discomfort that I want to get rid of by taking care of your so-called problem?

Conceptuality and the Mind

This leads to the mental quality, the quality of your state of mind.

Most of the time it seems that your state of mind is inside you, so nobody can see it, thank heavens. They don't really know what is going on. At the same time, your state of mind does affect what you do and what happens to whomever you are caring for. Of particular relevance is the notion of distractedness and the ability to steady your mind. It is a great help to be able to ground your mind a little bit, to learn how to hold your mind and to relax your mind on the spot. The phrase I like for dealing with your mind, particularly in situations that are painful, situations where there is suffering, our own and others, is "When the situation goes up, don't let your mind go up, and when the situation goes down, don't let your mind go down." The point is to develop a steadiness of mind.

One misconception about mindfulness is that it's just about being calm and collected all the time. I think that an overwrought description of meditative practitioners is that they are supposed to be smiley and nice all the time. But there is an insight aspect to working with mindfulness practice as well. The way I like to look at that is that it means not believing everything you think. The tendency, sadly to say, is that we actually do believe what we think. Most of the time we think that what we are perceiving is what is actually going on. We are not as cynical as we should be about our tendency to define things. We don't like things undefined, so we try to define things and we try to direct things. And it is my experience that you can't force situations. You can't force realization, you can't force someone to do things the way you want them to, you can't force healing, you can't force connectedness, and you can't force health.

We like to fix things, we like to make things happen, we want to figure out what to do. But more often than not, the thing to do is not to do anything. After not doing anything, we can do lots, but first we have to not do anything. First we have to be receptive. First we have to extend our antennae, we have to tune in. When I was in school they were always telling us how to cross the street. They'd say, "Stop, look, and listen." The idea was to keep us from getting run over. We get run over by a distracted mind, emotional upheavals, and just general panic. So if there is no other practice that you apply as you go about daily life, if you just go about the practice of stopping momentarily, just stopping, it's amazing what happens. Just stop.

As we are challenged, I think we tend to get speedier. We get more and more desperate to figure something out. We feel the responsibility of having to take care of the situation and having to be good at it, and along with that comes the fear of failure, the fear of mistakes. Those types of thoughts build and build, but at any point you can stop. You can stop. You can cut it. You can stop at any moment and start fresh.

Unifying Our World

Another aspect of healing that we can work with all the time is what you might call unifying our world—bringing into unity or harmony the mental swirling between what used to be happening, what should be happening, what might be happening, and collapsing all that into what actually is happening right now.

What Used to Be

If you are sick, there is a lot of feeling of what used to be. There is the notion that you can get back to "normal," but there is no normal to get back to. You can't go back to anything—you can only go forward. That is life: you can only go forward. And there is no normal. It is not un-normal to be sick, and it is not normal to be healthy. It is normal to be whatever is happening.

What Should Be

When we are not swirling around with what used to be, we are dwelling in what "should be." How many times do you think, "This is wrong. This should not be happening"? We have solid ideas of what should be happening in the world according to us. We think, "This is what should be happening—but it's not." So we get caught in the pain of being stuck with what is happening versus what we want to be happening. Not only what we want—what justice demands should be happening, but is not.

What Is

So where does that leave us? Nowhere. There is no alternate reality beyond what is actually taking place. Who cares what used to happen? Who cares what might be happening instead? None of that is in fact happening. What matters is what is, what we are confronted with this very moment. Whether you like it or not is beside the point. Instead of spinning out varieties of alternate scenarios, you could start by accepting what is currently happening and going from there.

The question then becomes: Now what? Can we connect with the situation as it is? Can we connect with another person as they are? Can we actually accept another person as they are in a situation as it is, without immediately trying to fix any of it?

This approach may sound defeatist. If you accept everything that is happening, it would seem that nothing is going to change. But when you reach the point where things are the way they are, and you acknowledge that, it is possible for a direction forward to arise from the connection between you and the other person, rather than from some preconceived notion or the desire simply to get out of an uncomfortable situation one way or another and then leave.

Lightness and Dynamism

I've also noticed the value of inquisitiveness, or taking an interest, and the value of tuning in to the freshness of each encounter. Even if you see the same person again and again, each encounter is new and each encounter is complete. The world is not inherently interesting or dull. It's up to you: if you take an interest, the world becomes interesting.

If you take an interest in the other person, and you pay attention to the small things like how he speaks, how she is in her body, you can infuse kindness and acceptance into the space you share. When you do so, you can feel the energy shift. We have much more power than we think to shift the energy through our presence and through our genuine interest in the other person.

This kind of interest comes along with a certain lightness of being. It's easy to lose track of that quality. It feels so very heavy to realize the amount of suffering people are dealing with at every level and in so many ways. Sometimes we find ourselves adding to the heaviness. We feel we should be heavy as a way of sympathizing with everyone else's heaviness because we think it will somehow show how empathic we are. "If I feel crappy, just like you do, that shows how much I care." I think that is a misunderstanding of what it is to be kind, healing, and compassionate.

It is possible to experience a quality of lightness in going through life, a lightness that comes from taking a big view of the endless turning of happiness and sadness, of suffering and relief, pain and pleasure, feeling lost and feeling found, sickness and health. Health is not fixed; we are constantly changing. We are never totally healthy and we are never totally sick. Instead, the interplay between health and illness is an endless cycle. And what we are doing in encountering one another is never the same from one instant to the next.

There is a dynamic happening, and it is a mistake to freeze it at any one point. To freeze it, end it, define it, or limit it. Instead we should aspire to place our interaction humbly within the great space of human experience. We could acknowledge our mutual vulnerability and challenges. We could open our hearts to our own vulnerability and be vulnerable together. To do so, we need to be willing to be wrong, willing to be un-knowing, willing to make mistakes—but it is all worth it. It is all worth it for at least one moment of connection. Within that connecting point, magic happens, healing happens, and people transform.

In healing others, we ourselves are healed, and in transforming others, we too are transformed. It is said that the garden grows the gardener. In the same way, the patient grows the caregiver. That is the way it works, even though we may think otherwise. That is the way it works.

Hospital Song

Rafael Campo

Someone is dying alone in the night.
The hospital hums like a consciousness.
I see their faces where others see blight.
The doctors make their rounds like satellites,
impossible to fathom distances.
Someone is dying alone under lights,
deficient in some electrolyte.
A mother gives birth: life replenishes.
I see pain in her face where others see fright.
A woman with breast cancer seems to be right
when she refuses our assurances
that we won't let her die alone tonight;
I see her face when I imagine flight,
when I dream of respite. Life punishes
us, faces searching ours for that lost light
which we cannot restore try as we might.
The nurses' white sneakers say penances,
contrite as someone dying in the night.
As quiet mercy, the morning's rites
begin. Over an old man's grievances,
his face contorted in the early light,
an aide serenely tends to him, her slight
black figure fleeting, yet all hopefulness—
her face the face of others who see light,
like someone dying at peace in the night.

Hospital Writing Workshop

Rafael Campo

Arriving late, my clinic having run
past 6 again, I realize I don't
have cancer, don't have HIV, like them,
these students who are patients, who I lead
in writing exercises, reading poems.
For them, this isn't academic, it's
reality: I ask that they describe
an object right in front of them, to make
it come alive, and one writes about death,
her death, as if by just imagining
the softness of its skin, its panting rush
into her lap, that she might tame it; one
observes instead the love he lost, he's there,
beside him in his gown and wheelchair,
together finally again. I take
a good, long breath; we're quiet as newborns.
The little conference room grows warm, and right
before my eyes, I see that what I thought
unspeakable was more than this, was hope.

Taking the Precepts as Your Guide: How to Approach Difficult Decisions, Accept the Consequences, and Not Keep Yourself Up All Night

8

CRAIG D. BLINDERMAN

An Ethical Dilemma: Request to Hasten Death

The Problem

Mr. Lewis, a lively and relatively high-functioning eighty-seven-year-old, requested that his pacemaker be inactivated. He explained to his primary care physician that he'd noticed a change in his cognitive functioning: forgetfulness and scattered thinking. His wife had died of vascular dementia approximately five years ago, and noticing some of her symptoms within himself was deeply troubling. Extensive neurologic evaluation determined that his objective neurologic functioning was not significantly impaired and that there was no other reversible medical explanation for his symptoms. There was concern, however, that this presentation may be a sign of underlying depression, an early onset of dementia, or a delirium that emerged following the placement of his pacemaker.

Mr. Lewis, his two adult sons, and their spouses felt strongly that his quality of life had declined so much, that his current state of health was so unacceptable to him, that he sought to end his life by deactivating his pacemaker and dying of subsequent congestive heart failure.

The Precepts

The Ten Grave Precepts

1. Not Killing
2. Not Stealing
3. Not Misusing Sex
4. Not Lying
5. Not Giving or Taking Intoxicants
6. Not Discussing Faults of Others
7. Not Praising Yourself While Abusing Others
8. Not Sparing the Dharma Assets
9. Not Indulging in Anger
10. Not Defaming the Three Treasures (Buddha, Dharma, Sangha)

The Ten Grave Precepts are what Zen students of the path vow to uphold when committing to practice together. These precepts provide an ethical structure for people living together in community and are also thought to be essential guidelines for one's own spiritual development.

While there are many ways to reflect on the precepts, I will focus primarily on the relational perspective: an inquiry into whether our thoughts and actions are useful, skillful, and in a compassionate spirit.

Unlike Aristotelian virtues, the precepts are not for the sake of building character or improving one's virtuous qualities. Rather, they allow us to move toward a life of right action. The precepts can be used to reflect on various aspects of our lives to see what motivates our behavior—are we speaking and acting from a place of compassion, or is our mind clouded by delusion or other beliefs?

This way of approaching the precepts, I believe, can offer us as healthcare practitioners an opportunity to reflect on whether our actions are in accord with the professional goals of medicine, nursing, chaplaincy, and other allied health professions. That is, are we acting out of compassion? Do we act to alleviate suffering? Are we focused on the healing of our patients? Can the precepts be used not as a means of "solving" a medical ethics dilemma, but as a way to better understand our intentions and attitudes in the process?

Not Killing

The literal perspective would simply not permit us from assisting in ending Mr. Lewis's life through the deactivation of his pacemaker. Though he has a right to discontinue life-sustaining treatment under US law, this ethical precept would nonetheless ask that we explore this request more deeply.

Thich Nhat Hanh interprets the precept in the following way: "Aware of the suffering caused by the destruction of life, I vow to cultivate compassion and learn ways to protect the lives of people, animals, and plants. I am determined not to kill, not to let others kill, and not to condone any act of killing in the world, in my thinking, and in my way of life."

Would agreeing to deactivate the pacemaker be an act of compassion, releasing the patient from what he believes to be an unacceptable quality of life? Are there other ways to reduce the patient's existential suffering than letting him die from heart failure? Surely this is the first "gut" reaction many have when they are asked to contemplate following through with this request. But does that mean that we can *never* discontinue a life-sustaining therapy when the discontinuation will lead to the patient's death? Of course, there are examples when the suffering and burdens of treatment outweigh any possibility for healing or for the patient's well-being. In such circumstances, the killing is not in the discontinuation but perhaps in the continuation of treatment. That is to say, we may be "killing" the memory or even the dignity of the patient through continued life-sustaining therapy. Or perhaps by maintaining the patient on life support we are "killing" potential moments of peace and healing for the patient and his family even as his body is dying. The contextual factors of time, degree, condition, and place obviously affect how we interpret this precept, moving from a literal interpretation of killing to an inquiry into "What is killing?"

According to the Zen Peacemakers, an organization of socially engaged Buddhists, "Recognizing that I am not separate from all that is. This is the precept of Non-Killing."

Not Stealing

This precept moves the angle of inquiry further from what we have explored above. That is to say, what might we be "stealing" if we were to honor the patient's request? Would we be robbing the patient and his family of potential moments of healing, love, and understanding? Would we be "stealing" opportunities for transcendence or awakening?

Another way in which we can be guided by this precept is when we consider our interactions with the patient and family. Are we fully present and attentive with the patient and family? Not listening and not being present may be thought of as "stealing" a potential moment of understanding and healing in our shared encounter.

We may also use this precept by asking ourselves, "How can I be satisfied with what exists? Can we help the patient and family be satisfied with the current conditions, or must we change something radically?" Dogen Zenji states, "The self and things of the world are just as they are. The gate of emancipation is open." Can we assist this patient and his family to accept what is, to be free from ideas about life, health, and death? Can we, ourselves, be free of such ideas?

Not Misusing Sex

The Zen Peacemakers offer a broader interpretation of this precept: "Meeting the diversity of life with respect and dignity. This is the precept of Chaste Conduct." Therefore, it is not sex itself, but its misuse—treating the other without respect and dignity—that is the true cause of harm.

How then can we respect Mr. Lewis? How can we approach him

with dignity? He presents his providers with a serious request to help end his life. He finds his current state of life unacceptable. Can we help bring dignity to his state of memory loss? Are there ways that he could be helped physically or socially to render the conditions of his current mental health less intolerable? Addressing his decline in functioning with respect and compassion may give him a sense that he is being listened to, that his suffering is real, and that it is *our* concern, as well as his.

Not Lying

One of the primary challenges in addressing any medical ethics case is assessing the medical "facts"—the likely prognosis, available treatment options, risks and benefits of the various treatment options, etc. Speaking honestly can be challenging when there is so much uncertainty. Without speaking falsely, how can we make recommendations to a patient when there is so much unknown? Much of medical knowledge is based on statistics, but statistical information can never be applied directly to the patient we are encountering. For that patient, the chances are either 0 or 1 that an event will happen, regardless of the chances of an outcome occurring in similar patients. Therefore, how can I know what I am stating is not false, or at least misleading?

The precept reminds us that we need to listen attentively and respond with a compassionate heart, transparent about the limits of medical knowledge. In doing so, we will be able not only to contribute our medical opinion, but also to respond from a place of understanding and intention to alleviate the patient's suffering, not from a false view that we actually know the outcome or the best course of action.

Not Giving or Taking Intoxicants

In the context of Mr. Lewis's case, this precept can be interpreted as avoiding anything that may delude the mind. Bodhidharma, the founder of Zen Buddhism, interprets the precept in the following way:

"Self-nature is subtle and mysterious. In the realm of the intrinsically pure Dharma, not giving rise to delusions is called the Precept of Not Giving or Taking Drugs."

We should avoid needing to be "right." This is a mistaken way of thinking that likely arises out of our notions of power, position, reputation, responsibility, etc. In any case, thinking that "we know what is best" for Mr. Lewis and his family is a kind of delusion—it means that our minds are not clear to other options, other possibilities, nor are we able to be fully empathic to the patient's existential suffering. Indeed, our desire to change the circumstances to "help" Mr. Lewis may itself be a deluded way of thinking, regardless of how laudable it may seem.

Can we see the situation clearly, in all its implications—for the patient, for his family, for his cardiologist, for his PCP, for the hospital, for the healthcare system? What sort of precedent would be set if we were to grant Mr. Lewis's request? What would it mean to deny his request? How can we see things more clearly in order that we might provide guidance to this suffering man and his desperate family?

Not Discussing the Faults of Others

Many of the healthcare providers involved in this case reflected on how difficult it was *not* to judge the patient's family for agreeing and even trying to facilitate the deactivation of the patient's pacemaker. Many felt that this was unduly influencing the patient's decision-making and autonomy.

The healthcare team could not truly know the family's motivations and intentions for their loved one. Nonetheless, several healthcare providers found fault with the family's decision to help Mr. Lewis end his life rather than finding other means of reducing his suffering. This natural inclination to find fault in others and, moreover, to discuss it in a healthcare team will likely create more distrust and separation between the treating team and the patient and family.

This precept challenges us to unconditionally accept whatever is given in each situation. In the case of Mr. Lewis, we should attempt to fully accept his family's position and their motivation to help him alleviate his suffering. Of course we need to remain open to all other possible motivations, but this will become clearer over time through direct clinical involvement, not through judging immediately upon hearing about the case.

This precept is of particular importance when there is significant conflict between the healthcare team and the family, or between family members and the patient, or any permutation of conflict that may arise in healthcare. Remaining open to—and not judging—the perspectives of all who are involved in the conflict is the first step toward finding a negotiated solution and respecting everyone who has a stake in the conflict's outcome.

Not Praising Self While Abusing Others

According to Buddhist teaching, there is no difference between self and other. This precept asks us to investigate how we separate ourselves from others—from our patients, from our colleagues, from our healthcare system.

This precept has particular resonance when it comes to medical error. In contemporary thinking about medical error, it is not *one* person's fault when something goes wrong, but rather the responsibility of everyone in the healthcare system that was part of the process (the physician prescriber, the pharmacist, the nurse, etc.). The precept supports this notion of collective or shared responsibility. We do not say, "I am blameless in this incident, it is he that is responsible." Instead, we each recognize that we are collectively responsible for the well-being of our patients.

Not Sparing the Dharma Aspects

This precept asks that we consider our generosity in all things. According to the Zen Peacemakers, the precept can be stated in the following way: "Using all of the ingredients of my life. This is the precept of Not

Being Stingy." We should inquire into whether we are withholding anything in our interactions and actions.

How can we live up to this demanding requirement? Are we holding back in our care for others? Are we too tired to listen attentively? Are we distracted in the moment when our patient most needs our attention and empathy? Being generous with our time and attention may give the patient a feeling of comfort and prevent feelings of abandonment or not being listened to.

How can we give generously to Mr. Lewis and his family? Perhaps we can start by fully appreciating his unique circumstances, listening attentively, offering words of comfort and reassurance, reframing misconceptions, giving our advice and counsel, offering to work together to find a solution that everyone can be comfortable with.

Not Indulging in Anger

It's easy to want to change reality, whether for the purpose of serving our patients or for our own lives. In letting things be as they are, we are less likely to engage in anger. Bodhidarma states this precept in the following way: "Self-nature is subtle and mysterious. In the realm of the selfless Dharma, not contriving reality for the self is called the Precept of Not Indulging in Anger."

When we seek to change reality we may become angry when it does not change according to our wishes. This is true whether the object we seek to change is a situation or a person's attitudes and actions. This precept asks us to look at how we may become angry. In the above case, we can easily find ourselves being angry with the patient's family. How could they support (and encourage) Mr. Lewis in hastening his death? We may believe that children and their spouses should behave or believe otherwise. Perhaps they should be trying to persuade Mr. Lewis *against* the desire to deactivate his pacemaker. Perhaps they should be asking themselves whether they are really acting in the patient's best interests.

Thoughts like these may anger us, but this is where the precept can guide us toward accepting a larger view of reality. By seeking to understand, through curiosity and compassion, we may be better able to empathize with their concerns and worries. Possible underlying issues may become manifest—a respect for Mr. Lewis's autonomy and dissatisfaction with his current quality of life, his underlying fear of disability and dependency, or his deep wish to avoid further suffering, etc. For Mr. Lewis, there may be the desire not to be a burden to others, to die on his own terms, to face the reality of cognitive disability with dignity, not dependency. All of these underlying interests may become clear if we can avoid anger and approach the reality of the situation as it is, with all the complex beliefs, desires, and fears that inform our decisions.

Not Defaming the Three Treasures

This last precept is perhaps the most abstract for a healthcare provider. What do we mean by defaming the Three Treasures or the Three Jewels of Buddha, Dharma, and Sangha? Sangharakshita, the founder of the Triratna Buddhist Community, interprets this precept in the following way: "I undertake the item of training which consists in abstention from false views." He also says, "Transforming ignorance into wisdom, I purify my mind."

Again, we are reminded of how precious this human life is—that we are a vehicle for perfecting wisdom and clarity of mind. In remembering this aspiration, we may be better able to approach this challenging ethical dilemma. In Mr. Lewis's case, members of our interdisciplinary team—physician, fellow, chaplain, and social worker, as well as the hospital's clinical ethicist—collectively spent many hours listening attentively and mindfully to both the patient's and his family's concerns and worries. Each member of the team approached the patient's distress and suffering in its totality, not as some problem to fix but as a shared responsibility. We attempted to abstain from false views through nonjudgmental listening, which proved to be the most effective way to connect with the patient and his family. We tried to see the family and patient, as well as ourselves, enmeshed in a web of suffering and responsibility.

In the end, our team managed to forgo previously held beliefs or biases in favor of a new understanding. We resisted proposing a solution, but instead attempted to understand and alleviate the underlying suffering of the patient and family. Integrating a deep belief in the inherent wisdom within each of us, we hoped to create a space of healing for all those involved in caring for this patient. By simply remembering why we do the work that we do, we can return to each case with a fresh perspective, free of delusion and judgment.

Working with the Precepts; Not "Solving" the Case

The precepts encourage self-reflection and help us see reality as it is, not as we would want it to be. Through carefully investigating how we *relate* to the ethical issue (or issues) at hand, we become more present and connected, allowing the unique circumstances to be seen for what they are. The use of biomedical principles and casuistry-based analyses are useful tools, but they do not necessarily resolve the inner struggle that we may feel when faced with an ethical dilemma, nor do they require that we see the interconnectedness of our lives and actions.

The struggle for me in this case was that I could intellectually rationalize the patient's right to discontinue a medical therapy regardless of whether it would hasten his death, but I felt that this was not something that I could suggest or perform in this circumstance. I attempted to connect more fully to the suffering than the stated request. The precepts help remind me to reflect on my attitudes and actions. Was I being open? Was I being intimate? Was I able to connect? Were notions of "right" and "wrong" preventing me from truly listening and being present? Could I exercise patience and skillful deliberation? Could I allow for a nonjudgmental, open space to offer what was needed?

After much deliberation and reflection, we explained to Mr. Lewis that we would not be able to discontinue his pacemaker at this time. Most of us felt that there were still other options to consider before determining that Mr. Lewis's suffering could not be alleviated, at which time the most compassionate thing to do would be to deactivate the pacemaker and allow him to die.

The social worker and I offered options to Mr. Lewis and his family—increased social support, change in living environment, psychotherapy, pharmacotherapy, and other ideas. Our suggestions were met with hostility and frustration. "He has a right to have his pacemaker turned off!" his daughter exclaimed.

Bodhidharma teaches that we should "not contrive reality for the self." Was that what I was doing? Was I contriving this patient's reality for what I believed was right? I noticed that I wanted things to be a certain way, and how painful and disappointing it was to be rejected. How does one transform this anger into acceptance? It doesn't happen quickly.

Through speaking with spiritual friends I started to loosen my grip on how I thought things should be. As an ethical consultant in my hospital as well as a palliative care physician, I often rely on my moral and professional judgments to suggest what ought to be, whether they are recommendations for symptom management or to resolve an ethical dilemma. This is what we typically do. However, the outcome we wished for—alleviation of this man's suffering and his family's distress through some transformative process—was not likely to happen. What occurred to me, both in the ethics committee discussion of this case and through the palliative care team's assessment, was that there was a deliberative, reflective, and committed process. I could appreciate the process and the intimacy that was created in our time together with the patient, his family, and one another, regardless of the outcome.

In the end, Mr. Lewis and his family decided not to pursue any of the options that we suggested, and they transferred to another hospital where the decision was made to discontinue the pacemaker. The patient survived for several hours after the pacemaker was turned off and received adequate medications to relieve his symptoms until he passed away.

I was deeply saddened when I learned of this outcome. I was also surprised to learn that the other hospital's ethics committee had reached a different conclusion. Once again I found myself feeling separate, distraught, and guilty of not doing more. It was natural to want to place blame on the other hospital's clinicians and their ethics committee. But I found that blaming was not a skillful means, especially if I wanted to truly not be kept up at night second-guessing our understanding, worrying that we had failed in some way, and finding fault with other colleagues who approached this patient's care differently. Thinking about these things results in no shift toward equanimity. If anything, I learned that it even manifested physically as a tightening of my face and neck, which may have reflected my tightened grip on my own understanding of how things should be. I felt that we approached this case openly and spoke the truth, as we experienced and perceived it. So does it matter that the outcome was not what many of us would have wanted?

The Zen Peacemakers interpret the Seventh Grave Precept as "Speaking what I perceive to be the truth without guilt or blame. This is the precept of Not Elevating Oneself and Blaming Others." I came to rely on this wisdom in the ensuing days, weeks, and months. When asked about this case, I would reply that we had dutifully and compassionately assessed the distress of this patient and his family and offered our services and our whole selves in the process. We cultivated a place of intimacy through the exploration of the request, understanding that the outcome would ultimately be largely out of our control.

I may often find myself disagreeing with others' assessments, wanting to change the patient or family situation, often discouraged by narrow views and conceptions about how to care for seriously ill and suffering patients. But therein lies the trap. When I become attached to my perspectives, I become more separate and stuck. The precepts can then serve as a reparative to this small-minded habit, like the cool water in a deep well—refreshing, nourishing, and sustaining.

Meditation Practice: A Practice of Dying 9

Joseph Goldstein

In many ways meditation helps us to understand and relate to death and dying.

The word for meditation in Pali is *bhavana*, which means mental development, or bringing forth. In meditation practice we develop or bring forth a certain mental strength, so that the mind is not easily moved by reactions of fear or anxiety about unpleasant things. The practice trains the mind to pay attention to what is happening in the moment, rather than being lost and carried away by trains of thoughts, fantasies, and reactions. We come to face and accept a whole range of bodily sensations, some of which can be very painful. We learn to sustain balance and equanimity with a wide range of emotions. From this place of strength and balance, the mind is able to be with fearful or difficult experiences with less wavering or agitation. It is likely that some of these difficult experiences will arise in the process of dying, and to the extent that we have developed an ability to be with them, there will be that much more balance and peace at the time of death.

Meditation practice also deepens our understanding of dying through a gradual refinement of our experience of impermanence. We all know with our intellects that things are changing. Our work is to know it from living it, from the inside out. There is an interesting and subtle progression in meditation practice regarding our perception of change. At first we are aware of different experiences after they have already arisen; we notice them in the middle of their lifespan. For example, we may become aware of a thought or sensation or emotion only after it has been there for some time. But as mindfulness gets stronger and our perception clearer, we begin to see objects more quickly, just at the moment of their arising. And when the practice deepens even further, then we can clearly experience the beginning, middle, and ending of phenomena. There is a growing understanding of momentary birth and death as we see thoughts, sensations, emotions, sounds, and images arise and pass away moment after moment. The distinctness and discontinuity of phenomena is experienced very closely and intimately.

Following this stage of seeing the arising and passing away, the perspective shifts once again until it is primarily focused on the dissolution of each object. At this time the mind is seeing a continual momentary vanishing of whatever arises. There is the very real sense of not having anything to hold on to because everything is disappearing so quickly. The power of this insight into dissolution is greatly enhanced by the awareness that not only are the objects of perception vanishing but also the consciousness that knows them. Even though we might have previously seen that objects come and go, there might still have been a real sense of *someone* who was observing it all, *someone* who was knowing. But now even the knower is continually dissolving and vanishing in each moment. There is a deep sense of dying, moment to moment. When we see that consciousness itself is part of this process of momentary change, it can feel as if the rug is pulled out from under us. There's no place to take a stand, there's no place for the sense of "I" to reside. The stage of dissolution is quite a powerful turning point in the practice and gives new meaning to our understanding of death and letting go.

Perhaps the most profound experience of dying that happens in meditation is the experience of nibbana, the unconditioned, because that is opening to something that is beyond this mind-body altogether. The Buddha described it as the deathless, because it is something that is not born and therefore doesn't die. Opening to nibbana is a dying to everything we know, because it is beyond the domain or realm of the ordinary mind and its objects. This death into the deathless has a tremendous transforming power because it is an opening to a reality beyond ourselves, from which perspective we have a more complete understanding of who we are and what this process of life and death is about.

The Washing of the Body

Nick Flynn

Blood carries oxygen & each muscle
hungers for it

a fluorescent stutters above your head
I don't understand then I do

gasp to gasp I hold your hand your hand
becoming air &

after a while we get hungry
we ride the elevator down & after a while

you stop

~

Marie: *What happens now?*
Nurse: *First we wash the body,*
then we send him downstairs.
Marie: *Can we be the ones to wash him—*
I mean, can the men?

~

Twenty years I've tried to write this
only to end up

this isn't it, this isn't it

here

~

Again:

your mother
as we came off the elevator her tears

her palm on your door

Marie tells us
a pure light filled the room tells us

we would be the ones
that we would be the ones to wash you

the door behind us closes

~

A year earlier (*or was it after?*) in Prague I'd
stood before a mural at the Jewish

cemetery, twelve

panels (*twelve?*), a body passed
from death bed to grave

one panel titled
the washing of the body

& three men stood around him
& each held a cloth

~

The light dimmed now   no one knows how
to begin

then one finds a pan & fills it   then one floats
a small bar of soap

one says   *I've never seen a body*
one says   *I've never touched one*

A dead one   one laughs   *He's still here*
one says

one calls you *sweetie*

we each take a cloth   *Billy,*
we're going to wash you now,

Billy, sweetheart

~

I tried to write about the blizzard
I got stranded
after we scattered your ash

my truck (*remember?*)—your tv, your
chair, your rug—in back   it never made it

to the city, I abandoned it all in
the snow

~

The hair on your thigh mats beneath
my hand

faint blue your lips   your nostrils caked
blood

one strokes your forehead
one spreads your toes

He's in good shape   one says
No wasting   one says

~

The ring on your finger   soap won't release it
it's almost too late
you can almost not hear

once we untie your johnny the ring is all
that isn't you

your back still warm where the blood
pools

one whispers   *Sweetie,*
we're going to roll you over now

10 Redefining the Metaphor for Dying

Ram Dass

I sit with people who are dying. I'm one of those unusual types that enjoys being with someone when they're dying because I know I am going to be in the presence of Truth. In our Western culture, although death has come out of the closet, it is still not openly experienced or discussed. Allowing dying to be so intensely present enriches both the preciousness of each moment and our detachment from it.

My dear friend Deborah was dying at Mount Sinai Hospital in New York. She was a member of the New York Zen Center, and every evening her friends from the center came to her hospital room to meditate. Doctors entering this hospital room were surprised to find it lit by candles and filled with the fragrance of incense and the deep peace of people in meditation. In this busy big-city hospital, this group of people meditating had redefined the metaphor for dying. You can create your universe anywhere you are. A hospital is merely a collective of beings who share a certain model about what it's all about. Each night her doctors entered the room more gently. Curing a disease of the body is not always an option, but healing from the soul level is always possible. In working with those who are dying, I offer another human being a spacious environment with my mind in which they can die as they need to die. I have no right to define how another person should die. I'm just there to help them transition, however they need to do it. My role is just to be a loving rock at the bedside.

Working with the dying is like being a midwife for this great rite of passage of death. Just as a midwife helps a being take their first breath, you help a being take their last breath. To be there fully requires being deeply grounded in compassion and love. Compassion, in this instance, is just both of you becoming who you are together—like the right hand taking care of the left hand.

When you are with someone who is dying, be there with them. All you have to give is your own being. Be honest. Meditate and become aware that the pain or confusion is, and here we are, in quiet equanimity. We all have limits of tolerance. Stay as clear and conscious as possible as someone nears death. Open to the unexpected. Open and stay centered. If you remain centered, your calm presence helps to free all those around you. Go inside yourself to that quiet place where you are wisdom. Wisdom has in it compassion. Compassion understands about life and death. The answer to dying is to be present in the moment. To learn to die is to learn how to live. And the way you do that is by living each moment—this one, now this one—just being here now.

The moment when the soul leaves the body is palpable and deeply profound. To share consciousness with a person who is dying, to be with them and help them die consciously, is one of the most exquisite manifestations of service. It is one role you may want to try out.

Acknowledging the Shadow 11

Rodney Smith

Behind the repressed darkness and the personal shadow—
that which has been and is rotting and that which is not yet
and is germinating—is the archetypal darkness, the principle
of not-being, which has been named the Devil, as Evil,
as Original Sin, as Death, as Nothingness.
—James Hillman

While we are dying we may not have the strength to hold our psychic defenses in place. The parts of ourselves that we have long avoided and feared often return. Waiting in the darkened recesses of our consciousness lies the shadow, the forbidden side of our character, created by our fears and resistances. The shadow expresses itself through such mental habits as impatience, low self-esteem, hatred, and lust. It is here that dying takes us; it is here that we can soften and open to our whole being.

A shadow is cast only where light is obstructed. The shadow within our consciousness is created when the light of our self-acceptance is smothered by self-criticism, abnegation, and dislike. Our delight with one aspect of ourselves defines in the same moment our disgust for the shadowed opposite part. Fear of our shadow has kept us from acknowledging it as part of ourselves. Subconsciously we have screened our mental responses, permitting access to the ones that we like and disassociating from the others. The result of employing our defenses against the shadow is a growing conflict between our ideal self-image and the reality of who we are. Aversion creates a tension that forces the shadow to the surface even as we despise its appearance.

The mind contains all possibilities. The entire continuum of mental states can manifest within us because the range of the mind is all-encompassing. Under the right conditions we are vulnerable to any given emotion or attitude. We can temporarily repress certain states of mind, but over time those same attributes will return in force. We attempt to hold these qualities at bay through a variety of defense mechanisms, but we eventually end up dealing with their energies in one way or another.

The emergence of the shadow suggests that our mental lives are not entirely under our conscious control. The shadow responds to our aversion by becoming more dominant, not less. Nothing can be eliminated from the mind by willful intentions. We can hide from these qualities and pretend they do not exist or suppress them in our unconscious, but their power and force are only multiplied by our inattention. The effect of this is that the more life is lived under the influence of the shadow, the more we attempt to discard it from our view.

Fracturing our mental lives—our thoughts, attitudes, and beliefs—into the good and the bad is the work of the shadow. This inward activity simultaneously leads toward external divisions as well. Life and death are polar opposites that form in the wake of the shadow's activity. Life is seen as the force of good, light, creation, and love, while death is cloaked in destruction, evil, and desolation. Having created this imaginary division, we pit one against the other. We fracture the original wholeness of life by demanding it to be only one way. The division is entirely mind-created. It is the splitting off of what we want from what we resist. Our conflict is internal, not external. We struggle with our fears and desires and project the resulting confusion onto the natural unity inherent in life.

Carl Jung once remarked that he would rather be whole than good. Perhaps he meant that when we attempt to be good we paradoxically force the emergence of evil within ourselves, but when we allow the coexistence of good and bad within our psyche, out of that wholeness goodness will naturally manifest. We think that if we do not keep a constant check on ourselves we might become the tyrant that we most fear. However, it is the checking itself that divides the world and leads to tyranny. Before our checking there is natural harmony and symmetry; afterward, however, the world becomes contentious and antagonistic. Our own mind creates this duality.

Separating Life and Death

One of the great divisions created from our shadow is the disjoining of life from death. Often dying patients do not acknowledge this separation and talk about "returning home." This is the beginning of unifying the two halves. Most of us find it difficult to rest comfortably with thoughts of death in the middle of good health. We see existence as the opposite of extinction. We then pit our existence against our extinction in a contest we are bound to lose.

The world is awash in images of this contest, this separation of life from death. We portray death as the robber of life, a phantom cloaked in black that waits in darkness to descend upon its victim. We would like nothing better than to sweep the streets clean of all suggestions of our mortality. Many doctors view death as a failure of their profession, as if we were meant to live forever. The status of physicians in a society indicates its aversion to death and dying. We elevate the rank of those who, we feel, protect us against the thing we most fear.

One of the reasons death is viewed as inimical to life is because it causes pain. Virtually everyone at some point suffers the loss of a loved one, and the grief that follows is one of the most difficult emotions to endure because it can rob us of our purpose to live. It leaves us feeling as if life is devoid of meaning. If everything is taken away in death, what sense does life make?

Death eliminates everything we now see. A person dies and the life force is gone with only a shell remaining. Death revokes life, removes it from view, and therefore stands in opposition to it. It is difficult to see life in any other way except through the presence or absence of its forms. There is happiness when life is here and pain when it is gone. Life is valuable, death is not. Everything of value stands in contrast to its absence.

Many religions teach that life and death are two forms of the same truth. This was one of the messages of Christ when he died on Friday and was resurrected on Sunday. Why did he wait two days before reappearing to the world? Surely he could have arisen from the dead immediately if he had wanted to. During that time there was an enormous outpouring of grief from his followers. His return demonstrated that their grief had been misplaced. He allowed his followers to dwell in their misrepresentation of death, hoping that their pain would eventually open them to the truth of who he was. The act of grieving over his body was a denial that he lived outside of the corporal form.

Separating what we can see from what we cannot is the first step in creating the shadow. What we see is familiar to us. We rest comfortably where we feel safe. What we cannot see is unknown and usually feared. We hold tightly to life because we are afraid of its absence, which we project as annihilation, the void, and nothingness. We think of nothingness as a desert or as the vacuum of space. The end of life terrorizes us, so we shove it out of view, away from our conscious awareness, and let it assume the form of the shadow.

But by pretending death does not exist, we have not eliminated it; we have only closed our eyes. Its presence is still felt in our reactions. Our fear and anger are an indication of the presence of the shadow. When we react, we know that the shadow is behind the activity, and one of our strongly held beliefs, attitudes, or self-images is being threatened. Fear and the need to protect our self-image lead to emotional outbursts, eruptions that happen so quickly that we never understand what led to them.

We fight the intrusion of the shadow by holding fast to who we want to be. The shadow contains what we fear we might become. We shove what we fear down below the level of our awareness into the unconscious and then attempt to live out only desired qualities. The unconscious, which contains the shadow, is not a separately sealed section of our minds. It is just that fear has eclipsed it from view.

The language of the unconscious can be confusing to our intellect. The imagery and intense emotions are fearful. Some of its messages seem to pertain to the life we are living, and others seem more rooted in our collective humanity. Our rational minds like ideas in nicely bundled thoughts that make historic sense. The rational mind and the unconscious are like two people who attempt to communicate but speak different languages. To the dominant rational mind the unconscious is neither predictable nor consistent. Its presence seems mysterious and dangerous. The emotional charge of its language can easily throw us off center.

The unconscious threatens us only because we misunderstand it. If we allow it to speak its own language without censuring it, we can begin to hear what it says. To understand the shadow without distorting it, however, we need to let go of the fear that surrounds it. Although we may not be able to understand it using our intellect, we can begin to feel its expression and open to its rich imagery. Then it will tell us its story. That story may be disturbing or confusing, but it is our story and part of ourselves.

I worked with Ellis, a hospice patient, who had a recurring nightmare about death. He tried everything to keep from having the dream, but night after night he found himself alone in a room with a dark and mysterious shadowy spirit. When the apparition would begin to approach him, he would run away in terror. He could feel the figure's intense stare even as he ran, and then he would wake up in a panic. The following night he would have the dream again. As we worked together over several weeks I suggested he personalize death by giving it a name and asking it questions. We role-played the parts several times. He began to read accounts about dying and developed a genuine curiosity and interest in what death was like. One night as the same dream unfolded, he stopped running and turned around to meet death. He said his interest in death in that moment was stronger than his fear.

As he turned toward death it vanished, and he never had the recurring nightmare again.

Ellis was able to develop interest in the thing he feared the most. When he gave death his attention, he began to allow it as part of his consciousness, and its horror diminished in the light of his understanding. Even after the dream disappeared, Ellis had to renew his commitment to face his shadow. But the success he had in befriending his death convinced him that he could work with his difficulties.

But the shadow is a shadow only because of the power we give it. In the final evaluation neither the shadow nor its offspring, death, has ever been the problem. It is our aversion to what we think the shadow says about us that creates our desire to escape its message. Resisting death, we hold tightly to life. Our endless striving to avoid the shadow leads us to react to both living and dying. We desire the one and fear the other, thereby creating an inherent tension in which there is neither enjoyment of life nor understanding of death. Holding death at arm's length, we end up resisting life to the same degree.

The Meeting of Life and Death

Many patients who are dying no longer belong to a world that is fractured into life and death. When we know we are approaching the end of our lives we can no longer sustain our usual denial of death. Hospice patients who have this knowledge realize it is time to withdraw their energy and focus from the living. Sometimes there is a period of withdrawal in which patients will turn away from social interaction and move deeply into themselves. They will frequently come out of that period more remote and removed from family and friends. Their whole view may have shifted so that they now seem to live between two worlds rather than fixed exclusively in this one. Sometimes a patient will look through the person in front of him and attempt to communicate with people who cannot be seen. He will often gaze past this world and rest upon something or someone distant and hidden. It should be noted that these visions are not frightening to the patient.

In fact the opposite is true; they seem to offer the patient reassurance and comfort.

Medically, these perceptions are caused by a decrease in the circulation of oxygen to the brain and a change in the body's metabolism. But this physical explanation is only a partial one. For anyone who has seen a person go through these reality shifts, it is clear that this other world is as real to him as this one is to us. He is not hallucinating. We cannot dismiss what we witness with a medical banality merely because we cannot reference those same perceptions.

More to the point, the patient's view becomes more holistic when she no longer divides life and death into separate camps but indeed experiences them as a seamless continuum. When the patient frees herself from that false division, she may gain access to unseen worlds, worlds that would be available to all of us were we not so intent on fracturing this one.

Margaret was an elderly woman dying of breast cancer. When hospice first became involved, Margaret claimed that death was the absolute end and nothing existed beyond it. As she became more confined to her bed, Margaret would spend increasingly long periods by herself. Normally she was an extroverted woman, and her sudden desire for isolation concerned her family. As she became weaker she started to go in and out of a coma. The family noticed she would move her lips in silent speech to unseen people while she was in a semicomatose state. Once the hospice nurse gently called her name while she was in one of these states. "Margaret, Margaret, can you hear me?" The patient, focusing on something beyond what the nurse could see, looked through her and replied, "Margaret is not here right now. Her friends have come to take her away. She'll be back soon." A few minutes later her eyes were clear, and she spoke to the nurse about "going home." Two hours later she died very peacefully.

The question is how do we face our shadow? Do we divide the whole into opposing parts, creating a multitude of problems including the struggle between life and death? If we were able to discard part of our minds the solution would be simple. We could get rid of the shadow and live happily ever after. But obviously there is no way to eliminate any part of our consciousness. Even to think that the shadow could be extracted from the rest of the mind implies a misconception about its origin. The shadow exists only because we want life on our own terms and are unwilling to accept it as it is.

We see this in our ideas of good and evil and the suffering created from this division. If we look closely, we will see that evil is built upon our need to guard against further pain. When we suffer we pull back, separate, and protect ourselves against any intrusion. Hostility, rage, selfishness, dishonesty, and most other "negative" qualities are the result of insulating ourselves from our hearts. We think the way to heal is to keep everything at bay as if we needed fortification from further attacks. It becomes the world against us. It is light against dark. We become our own worst enemy.

As we learn from reflecting on death, we can use a different strategy to reclaim our nature and begin to heal. This lesson is not limited to the dying; the message is equally appropriate to the healthy. The reconciliation needed is for both sides of our character to coexist within the whole of our consciousness. Like the dying patient who heals himself by no longer warring against death, we also need to stop living a struggle we have created with our imagination. We end our suffering when we understand that we are diminished as human beings when any part of our character is denied. It is not a matter of being good or bad but of being complete and total. We have it all, why not be it all? Anything less forces the shadow to rule from behind the scenes.

The tapestry of existence is woven of many strands. Our character expresses the entire range of mental qualities manifesting in each moment. We are only what we are right now: no more, no less. No other side of our character lurks in the background waiting for an opportunity to take control, because that other side is part of our life in this moment as well. Everything can be dealt with here and now. Being whole means honoring all of these manifestations in the present. Once this is done, the energy that we put into maintaining our separation becomes available for more creative endeavors. Life and death return to their original unification.

Kendall was a hospice patient who was at war with his own history. He had mentally and physically abused his wife and daughter throughout much of their life together. Kendall had been an alcoholic for forty years. On the suggestion of his doctor in order to avoid further complications, he was still given alcohol throughout his illness. As he began to deal with his dying, his family could frequently hear him sobbing alone in his room. He hated the person he had become and lived with an enormous guilt and fear of his temper and rage. Kendall spent long sessions with the hospice chaplain seeking self-forgiveness and praying for forgiveness from God. Even in the midst of this self-degradation he would still fall into a hostile rage if his family made a simple mistake in his care. These outbursts would eventually propel him into further self-torment.

Unexpectedly, Kendall suddenly fell into a deep coma. Everyone thought he was dying and made all the necessary arrangements. Three days later he woke up and was completely alert and responsive. After a short period of time, everyone who knew him realized something had changed. The anger had disappeared, and he seemed more relaxed and less self-deprecating. When the chaplain asked him about these differences, he said he was tired of hating himself. He said he had to pull all parts of himself together to face his dying.

To paraphrase Abraham Lincoln, "A mind divided against itself cannot stand." Kendall understood he had enough difficulty facing his death without the additional burden of self-hatred. Who knows what happened to him while he was in a coma? The point is that he came out of this reverie with a strong sense of personal integration and a diminished shadow.

Dying teaches us that we will not be engulfed by evil if we permit the dark side to share time and space with the good. We see contentment expressed by many of those near death. Their message is that basic goodness lies in our wholeness, not in our struggle against evil. The goodness that manifests from the absence of conflict has no opposite. When something contains everything there can be no force aligned against it. It stands without opposition, rightly integrated.

Reflection and Exercise: The Shadow

Reflect on the enormous range of behavior and emotion within yourself and recognize that in response to every news story you could say, "There, but for the grace of God, go I." With similar birth conditions and life circumstances, you could be the thief or the heroine, the person with AIDS or the homeless. Reflect on the range of your own emotions, on how whimsical or circumstantial they can seem. If you were provoked in the right situation, is there any activity or emotion beyond your own potential to feel, think, or do?

Bring to mind a time when people you know have been thoughtful and have acted with good intentions. Feel how easy it is to care about and open your heart to them. Now bring to mind criminals and their crimes. Watch your heart close toward the rapist, murderer, and thief and recognize that their hearts are also closed. They acted out of their own suffering and perpetuated their pain in a chain reaction that has now closed your own heart. Feel the energy you expend to keep such people out of your life. Can you begin to open to even this kind of human suffering? Can you see such people as worthy of your caring even if they are deserving of punishment?

Reflect upon the changing intensity and quality of your emotional life. Emotions are not static conditions but fluctuating states of mind. What is actually contained within an emotion such as happiness? How long does it usually last? What conditions need to be present for happiness to manifest? How much control do you actually have over your emotions?

Choose any attitude or emotion that you experience often, such as anger or sexual desire. Over the next few days, try to notice the fluctuations in intensity of this state of mind. If you choose anger, for example, become aware of your feelings of annoyance, frustration, irritability, hostility, and rage. Notice how you relate to these variations in energy and activity. When do you lose your self-awareness? Are these feelings uncomfortable? Do you identify with all aspects of the emotion or only a certain range of its intensity? Feel the most uncomfortable part of the emotion. Can you allow it to be in your consciousness without acting it out?

Reflect on Carl Jung's statement that he would rather be whole than good. What does this mean to you? Think about a time when you were self-righteous. How did that feel? Was there a feeling of separation and distance from others? If you acted out or verbalized your feeling of self-righteousness, what consequences did it have? Reflect on what it means to be whole and complete without emphasizing any quality at all.

Choose a personal quality that you are proud of, such as your kindness, humility, or courage. Select a quality that you strongly identify with and that makes a clear statement about who you are. How do you feel when this quality expresses itself in action? Now look at its opposite: your anger, arrogance, or weakness. How do you feel when this opposite quality arises? Watch the arising and passing of both of these states. Now attempt to exclude the opposite quality entirely. Watch it over time and see what happens. Can it be done? What happens to the positive quality as you try to exclude the negative? What does this tell you about the nature of the mind?

Reflect on polar opposites, seeing how one defines the other.
How would you know one side existed without the other? Can you see opposites as different ends of the same continuum rather than as two separate qualities? Take any pair, such as worthiness and unworthiness, or likability and unlikability. Where would you put yourself along a continuum between the two? Reflect on the struggle to maintain your likability or self-worth when your inward life is always changing.

Choose any pair of opposites and investigate it for one week. For example, observe your tendencies toward honesty and dishonesty, generosity and selfishness, or clarity and confusion. Study both tendencies and see how you attempt to strengthen one at the expense of the other. Keep reminding yourself of their relativity: no matter where you are on the scale, there is more to achieve. Are you ever kind or generous enough? Is there any rest or contentment when you evaluate yourself in this way? Rather than attempting to strengthen one of the opposites, bring both within you. Bring your striving into awareness as well. Be vigilant of the full range of qualities along the scale without judging yourself by the presence or absence of any quality at all. Now step off the scale and allow all measurements to end.

Senryu

Bitter winds of winter—
but later, river willow,
open up your buds.

Becoming (and Sustaining) the Bodhisattvas We Already Are

12

Michael Kearney and Radhule Weininger

Becoming a healer means remembering who you already are. In Buddhist thought this is referred to as "realizing our Buddha nature." While this has implications for how we see ourselves as caregivers, it also affects how we see our patients, how we act in clinical situations, and how we practice self-care. Tibetan Buddhist teacher Chögyam Trungpa writes in *The Sanity We Are Born With*:

> According to the Buddhist tradition, people inherently possess Buddha-nature; that is, they are basically and intrinsically good. From this point of view, health is intrinsic. That is, health comes first: sickness is secondary. Health *is*. So, being healthy is being fundamentally wholesome, with body and mind synchronized in a state of being which is indestructible and good. This attitude is not recommended exclusively for patients but also for the helpers and doctors. It can be adopted mutually because this intrinsic basic goodness is always present in any interaction of one human being with another.

Seeing that our deepest nature is goodness and health allows us to be in the presence of suffering without burning out or drowning in despair.

The Nature of Suffering and the Nature of Healing

In April 2007, Balfour Mount and his colleagues Pat Boston and Robin Cohen published a research paper called "Healing Connections: On Moving from Suffering to a Sense of Well-Being." Working with a group of individuals living with terminal disease they asked, "What makes the difference between those who live their final months with what they themselves consider to be good quality of life, and are able to say that they are happy and that their lives have meaning, and those who, despite similar life circumstances, describe themselves as scared, lonely, unhappy, who experience their lives as meaningless and their quality of life as awful?"

To answer these questions they interviewed twenty-one individuals who were equally matched for all the demographics of age, sex, disease status, symptom burden, and socio-economic status. Half of the group appeared to be thriving and happy despite their terminal illness, while the other half appeared to be miserable and unhappy. Using a qualitative research methodology, they interviewed each person and analyzed their results to try to identify differentiating factors.

Their findings can be summarized quite simply: *What makes all the difference is the presence or absence of what they call "healing connections."* They identified four key areas in which these healing connections can occur. The first is with ourselves (for example, being happy and at peace in oneself); a second is with other humans; a third is with the phenomenal world (for example, with music or in nature); and finally, there are healing connections with what they called "Ultimate reality, however this was understood by that individual" (while some spoke of God, others spoke of love, and so on). When individuals experienced healing connections in any (it may have been one or more) of these areas, they described their quality of life as good and their lives as meaningful. In contrast, when individuals did not experience healing connections in any of these areas, they described their quality of life as poor and their lives as meaningless.

The individuals in this study, living in the final weeks and days of their lives, are offering us answers to the same existential questions that Siddhartha Gautama asked about the nature of suffering and the nature of healing.

Suffering as a Place of Healing

The bodhisattva is one who chooses to reenter the world of suffering again and again and again for the sake of all beings. It could be said that the bodhisattva's path into wholeness is suffering. In Western civilization we call this figure "the wounded healer," the one who knows from experience that suffering, their own and others, is a place of healing.

We have learned a great deal about the dynamics of the wounded healer from Buddhist scholar and environmental activist Joanna Macy. She teaches a powerful process for encouraging compassionate action on behalf of others and our world that she calls "The Work that Reconnects." There are four steps in the spiral of The Work that Reconnects. The first is gratitude, grounding ourselves in the heart so we have the courage to take the second step of "honoring our pain for the world." This is the pivotal move in the process, for as we honor our pain for the world, which Joanna describes as turning toward, leaning into, and allowing ourselves to experience our feelings of suffering, something quite unexpected happens. She describes this in the following way in an interview on *On Being*:

> We are called to not run from the discomfort and not run from the grief or the feelings of outrage or even fear and that, if we can be fearless, to be with our pain, it turns. It doesn't stay static. It only doesn't change if we refuse to look at it, but when we look at it, when we take it in our hands, when we can just be with it and keep breathing, then it turns. It turns to reveal its other face, and the other face of our pain for the world is our love for the world, our absolutely inseparable connectedness with all life.

She describes this as a "Tantric flip": as we allow ourselves to experience our pain for others, we "flip" into a realization of interconnectedness. This flip alters our perspective and brings us to the third step in the spiral process: "seeing with new eyes." We are in the same world but seeing it in a different way; things look different than before. Realizing our kinship with all life, we long to act to relieve the suffering of others and so, in the fourth and final move in this process, we "go forth" in compassionate action. Here is what this looks like at the bedside:

Joseph was in his early twenties and hospitalized with a severe acute exacerbation of chronic abdominal pain. Palliative care was consulted for recommendations with pain control and to offer him emotional support. His medical situation was very complex. He had been diagnosed with diabetic gastroparesis and the so-called "narcotic bowel syndrome." We were told, before ever meeting with him, that on no condition was he to have any opioid analgesics as these were exacerbating rather than helping his pain. He had been prescribed opioids over the years for his pain before it was diagnosed for what it was. By this time he had become dependent on them. His life was at a standstill because of his condition and the repeated hospitalizations this necessitated. He had lost his job, and his marriage was under a lot of strain.

When I (Michael) arrived on the floor to see him, I reviewed his chart and spoke with his primary care team. By then it was clear to me that any treatment options I might have suggested had already been considered and explored, all to no avail. I had already received calls from both his gastroenterologist and psychiatrist reiterating that it would be disastrous were I to recommend opioids.

I knew that I was walking into an impossible situation. As I approached his room I was at a feeling of loss. Just before opening the door I paused, took a deep breath, and made a short *bodhichitta* prayer that I often say to myself at moments such as this, "May all beings be happy." I knocked and went inside.

Before I finished introducing myself, Joseph interrupted me and said, "I know the narcotics are making things worse, but when this pain comes on bad I just want to die." I pulled over a chair and sat by the side of his bed and asked him to tell me about what had been happening. I listened as he told the story of his multiple admissions and the many hospitals he had been in, of investigations, of surgeries, of dashed hopes, and of the relentless return of the pain. He spoke of how he knew he was now seen as "drug-seeking" and of how his admissions through the ER had become a traumatic nightmare of pain and judgment. He finished by looking directly at me and saying, "How can you doctors not give someone the one thing that can relieve their suffering? How can you allow someone to continue suffering when you know you have something you could do that could bring them relief? I don't need narcotics at home. But when I have a pain crisis that brings me to the hospital, I have to have something to help me. And they are the only thing that works."

As I listened to Joseph I became aware that I was feeling very conflicted. I was deeply moved by his story of suffering and his anxious pleas for help. I wanted to respond, to give him what he was asking for, to make him better, to ease his suffering. And yet I knew I could not do that; I was not able to give him the one thing he wanted from me. I was feeling very uncomfortable. I wanted to get up and leave.

For many years I have been helped in my clinical practice by the image of "the wounded healer," one who chooses to stay, at times such as this, with her or his own pain and sense of impotence. Again and again I have seen how doing this, while continuing to be present in a heartfelt way to the other who is suffering, can awaken that individual's own healing potential. Recently, Joanna Macy had inspired me to deepen this practice and given me a way of understanding this in terms of the dynamics of compassion and interconnectedness.

As I sat there listening to Joseph's story, aware of my pain in the face of his suffering and aware of my inability to do anything to make it better, I remembered the wounded healer, and I remembered Joanna's teaching. This gave me the encouragement to "hang in there" despite my feelings of discomfort and inadequacy.

I also remembered a short meditation process Radhule had recently developed for just such an occasion as this, one that she calls "The Compassion in Action Process":

1. In the face of the other's suffering, bring your attention inward and downward into the body.
2. Notice your physical experience, what is happening right now, in your body, and where.
3. Bring your attention to your breath and exhale gently to relax.
4. Notice your emotional experience, what feelings are there, and where.
5. With the exhale, allow yourself to drop down into the felt-sense of your experience and to linger there for just a little while: "suffer your suffering."
6. Offer compassion to yourself while continuing to breathe gently, holding this experience in your heart.
7. When you are ready, once again direct your attention outward and turn toward the other, noticing what you are feeling and what you are seeing.

As I brought my attention inward and down into my body, I noticed that my jaw was tightly clenched and that I was feeling achy. Then I brought my attention to the movement of my breath, and in particular to the sensations of the gentle release of the outbreath. I noticed that attending to the exhale in this way allowed me to relax, to loosen, to let go a little. Next, as I attended to what I was feeling about Joseph and his situation, I became aware of a mix of many different emotions. There were feelings of frustration and helplessness at not being able to alleviate his pain, as well as some anxiety about how he was going to react when he realized this, and shame at appearing a failure to my colleagues. At the same time, there were feelings of deep sorrow for this man and his young family who were trapped in such a miserable situation. As I recalled the "pivotal move" in this process, I consciously gave myself permission to drop into the felt-sense of what I was experiencing. There were sensations of rawness and aching around my heart. Though it was uncomfortable to do so, I deliberately chose to let my awareness drop into these sensations, allowing myself to experience what I was experiencing.

After a few moments, I remembered that the next step was to offer compassion to myself. I immediately knew that this would not be easy. I was feeling like a failure, and I could not readily access a sense of warmth or kindness toward myself. Instinctively, I put my hand on my heart and became aware of the gentle sensations of pressure on the wall of my chest. As I did this, images came into my mind's eye of myself as a doctor. I saw myself arriving at my workplace prepared to do what I could to relieve the suffering of others, day after day, year after year. From the silence of my heart words came: "For the sake of all my relations, may I hold myself with gentleness and care." With this, a deep sigh swept through me. I continued to breathe gently while holding this experience lightly in my heart as I observed how my body was breathing, spontaneously, effortlessly, without my volition or control. For a few breaths I followed the gentle flow of the breath in this way. As I did so, I recalled words that had come to me earlier that day in my morning's meditation, "May all that is connected breathe us deeply well . . . May all that is connected breathe us deeply well . . ."

It seemed that allowing myself to experience my feelings of frustration and sorrow for Joseph had unlocked something. A knot in my heart had loosened. I felt my chest expanding and my jaw soften. The deep helplessness and hopelessness I had felt gave way to something that was subtle and hard to name. While there was something timeless about this experience, as I brought my attention back to the here and now and to Joseph sitting before me, I realized that it had only taken a minute or so. And yet even in that short time something essential had come back into balance. Something important had fallen back into place. A wave of warmth and concern for Joseph swept through me. As I listened to him finish speaking, I felt appreciation for his courage and resilience. I expressed my heartfelt gratitude to him for sharing his story with me. Our eyes met. In the silence of that moment I knew that the conversation had just begun.

Sustaining the Bodhisattva with "No-Self-Care"

There are three well-recognized syndromes of occupational stress. *Burnout*, which arises from the stresses generated between the individual and institutional or bureaucratic processes, resulting in chronic emotional and physical exhaustion, a sense of never quite achieving one's goals, and feelings of being increasingly detached and disconnected from others and one's work. What is sometimes called *Compassion Fatigue* (which from a Buddhist point of view is a misnomer; compassion does not fatigue but rather replenishes us) is more accurately termed *secondary traumatic stress disorder*, as it describes the effects of being secondarily or vicariously traumatized by another's suffering. This can lead to the symptoms of post-traumatic stress disorder. Thirdly, there is *Moral Distress Syndrome*, which occurs when one knows the correct action to take but is powerless to do so. This may result in either the symptoms of burnout or compassion fatigue/secondary traumatic stress disorder, or a mixture of both.

Existing models of self-care operate on the assumption that there is a "self" to take care of. What might be described as the traditional model of self-care advocates having good professional boundaries as protection from the stresses of the workplace and an effective program of rest and renewal on leaving work—cultivating what is referred to as "a healthy work-life balance." If we were to use a water metaphor for occupational stress, then feeling overwhelmed by work stresses might be seen as "being flooded" or "being underwater," and the classic approach to self-care as holding one's breath (having good professional boundaries) and coming up for air (having recreational activities outside of the workplace).

Some newer approaches to self-care emphasize the value of clinician self-awareness or mindfulness. There is an increasing body of data to show that self-awareness is itself protective. Self-awareness can enable the clinician to be highly present, sensitively attuned, well-boundaried, and, most important, heartfelt to another who is suffering in even the most stressful of situations, in a way that allows the clinician to receive as well as give in the clinical encounter, a process that has been called "exquisite empathy."

Clinicians describe how they emerge from such encounters feeling replenished rather than depleted. Furthermore, self-awareness allows for self-monitoring. For example, if something has triggered a reactive cascade of feelings and an urge to act out, self-awareness enables one to metaphorically press a "mindful pause button" and consider a range of possible options. The clinician can then discern what is most appropriate to this person in these circumstances and choose to respond skillfully and with compassion. While self-awareness involves innate cognitive skills and processes, it can be further developed through four distinct approaches: self-knowledge ("clinician know thyself"), self-empathy (or self-forgiveness), mindfulness (purposeful and nonjudgmental attentiveness to one's own experience, thoughts, and feelings), and contemplative awareness (the awareness that one's encounters with others are embedded in bigger and deeper fields of relationships).

Self-awareness allows us to meet the one who suffers with heightened presence, sensitivity, and accuracy. With self-awareness we know both the limits of what we can give and when it is appropriate to be present to the one we care for with a full and open heart. In terms of the water metaphor of occupational stress, self-awareness allows us to breathe underwater as we find regeneration and renewal in the work itself.

We would like to propose a third approach to self-care: "no-self-care." The core assumption here is that there is not a self to take care of—or, at least, that there is not a self in the sense we usually think of it. The Buddhist concept of *anatta* refers to the emptiness of the concept of self, to "no-self," but not in a nihilistic sense. The "no-self" of anatta means "no-solid-separate-permanent-self." There is self but it is self in relationship—self as part of a much bigger framework and process. This has important implications for how we see ourselves as healers, how we understand healing, and for resilience in the workplace. The "no-self" of anatta means that the healer I already am is fluid, interconnected, and ever changing—that healing is not something that I personally do to or for another. Healing is what naturally happens when we (the other and I) become part of the fluid, interconnected, impermanent, always-changing process that is ultimate reality.

So it is no longer a matter of congratulating ourselves when things go well or blaming ourselves when they don't. We do our best. We contribute to the process. Then something happens that is, ultimately, not in our control. What *is* in our control is to set our intention, choose to do what we think is in the best interest of the other, and let go of the outcome. Aware of the interconnectedness of all things, we cultivate the conditions for healing within ourselves and in our relationship with the suffering other. Then, together, we wait to see what emerges.

What then might "no-self-care" look like? If the primary move in traditional models of self-care is to establish good professional boundaries, and if the primary move in newer models of self-care is the cultivation of self-awareness and mindfulness, the primary move in no-self-care is what we call "deep connection practice"—practices that bring us into an experience of self as fluid, porous, permeable, dynamically interconnected, and mutually coarising in what is, as our indigenous brothers and sisters remind us, "a world of relatives." We can think of deep connection practices as being either "inner" or "outer" depending on where the primary object of our attention is located. Mindfulness of breathing is one example of an "inner" deep connection practice, whereas time in nature is an example of an "outer" deep connection practice.

We each need to discern and customize deep connection practices that work for us. In terms of the water metaphor, we might think of these practices as "breathing holes," those holes in the ice that seals work hard to keep open during the Arctic winter so that they can move from the frozen world above to their food source below and so that they, and others, have somewhere to breathe. We each need "breathing holes"—places, people, and practices that allow us to move from the frozen world of isolation to the fluid world of relatedness, and that allow us to emerge when necessary and fill our lungs with clear, replenishing air.

Here are some possible questions to reflect on to enable you to identify your own deep connection practices:

- What makes me feel most awake, alive, connected?
- What brings me into a lightness of being and a peace of heart?
- What brings me into gratitude?
- What brings me into a sense of deep belonging?
- What awakens my longing to care for all beings?
- When, where, and doing what do I think, "I am glad to be doing this for my great-grandchildren?"

To sustain the bodhisattvas that we already are, we need self-knowledge, self-empathy, and mindfulness, each in the context of ongoing deep connection practices, and always in the spirit of *bodhichitta*, the mind of enlightenment, motivated by compassion for all beings.

Appointment

Jason Shinder

When I visited the doctor, I am reminded that I, too, was sick.

And still am. Not because of sadness or because in 1976
I wasn't kind to my father at his deli on Kings Highway,

Brooklyn. I swept the floor without talking to him, without

knowing what work was. And money. When I looked,
he was slumped in a chair, pulling the ends of his mustache.

I'm not sick because of anything; just because. The doctor

digs his fingers into the liquid tumors growing just beneath
the skin of my neck and in the crossword puzzle of hair

under my armpits; I imagine the yellow leaves hanging

from the branches of a willow tree that fall in Paris long ago.
A young Chinese nurse stands in the doctor's office, alone

in her body as if under a streetlamp, the white neon light

of her breath going out of her, going out. I slip my pants below
my knees. When I was in love I could not get used to the hours

with someone in them. What have you been feeling? Doctor asks.

Nothing. I turn away and cough, and, in that moment, when
the doctor is feeling my grainy-skinned quiet pair of balls

in that precise and careful way, I am ashamed that something

in me, some absence about myself, some loneliness I've never
understood, which sometimes disappoints, but which sometimes

shows me who I am, is made better by his slight touch.

Afterbody

Jason Shinder

After the chemo and the throwing up,

after the passion of a life upset,
after I watch the color of the skin turn yellow—

my thoughts more and more about things

that never happened—after I spent many nights
alone, happy for the police dramas on television,

I kept to myself.

The cancer saved me from having to go
to another book party

from having to ask Mr. M to come back

who, after all, had fallen out of love
because I was different now, thin,

bone and severity, free to consider

my absence, where nothing aches
and the messy sexual hungers are far off

in the past. After I slept for days,

after the dazzle of wild, repeatable dreams,
there was no afterlife,

just the same way from the bed

to the bathroom and back again
without the body.

Untitled

Jason Shinder

If there is no cure, I still want to correct a few things

and think mostly of people, and have them all alive.
I want a door opening in me that I can enter

and feel the clarity of evening and the stars beginning.

One after another, I want my mistakes returning
and to approach them on a beach like a man

for whom there is no division between one way or another.

My most faithful body, you are not in the best of shape,
far from the glitter of the river in which you once swam.

But I want good tears when I stand on the street

and, from the sky, drifts down the finest mist on my face.
Not everything is given and it should not permit sadness.

Let me
Let me keep on describing things to be sure they happened.

13

The Raw Spot

Norman Fischer

One day in January, feeling expansive and cheerfully open to being interrupted, I picked up the ringing telephone in my study. Sherril was on the line. "Alan just died in Baltimore," she said. "Can you come over right now?"

Alan is Sherril's husband and my closest friend. We'd known each other forty years, since our days as students at the University of Iowa Writers Workshop, through years of Zen practice, through Alan's becoming a rabbi, my ordaining as a Zen priest, our establishing a Jewish meditation center together, through retreats, teaching sessions, workshops, marriages, divorces, children, grandchildren. We had shared so much for so long that we took each other's presence in the world as basic.

At first you don't know how to think about it. You are bewildered. What just happened? I had co-led a retreat with Alan earlier in the month, and we'd parted company just eight days before he died while walking on a country lane one bright morning. He had been so completely present at that retreat, and now he was—or so they told me—just as completely absent. What to make of this?

Of course I could say—and have often said—many things about such losses. Alan and I had frequently taught together about death and dying and loss and grief. It was a subject both of us had been concerned with most of our lives. The Buddhist teachings on death and dying are very familiar to me, as are the many associated practices and reflections. It's not that such practices and thoughts were not with me during the days and weeks after Alan's death; they certainly were, and they made my experience of loss much more solid and poignant. But I had always known that these teachings do not explain anything or fix anything or armor you against pain. They only clear the ground for what there is to be felt at the time of a loss. They help you to feel what I felt: the supreme oddness, sorrow, and joy of our lives. We are here. We are gone. All dharmas are empty of own being, there is no coming no going, no increase no decrease, no birth, no death, no suffering, no end of suffering. So the Heart Sutra says. The Diamond Sutra says that all conditioned things are to be viewed as dreams, flashes of lightning, bubbles, dew drops, magic shows. Still, tears come. There's no contradiction.

In the days and weeks that followed Alan's death, I spent a great deal of time with Sherril and their children and with Alan's siblings, who'd come from back East for the funeral. Alan had been the rabbi of a large congregation in San Francisco and had been connected to many other meditation and social action communities, so there was an outpouring of love and support from many people. I received cards and emails from all over the world. And I was really grateful that I could cry with others when I felt like crying, and I could feel so much love for so many people who also loved Alan. Loss does that: it wounds the heart, causing it to fall open. Love rushes into and out of the opening, love that was probably there all along, but you didn't notice it because you were too busy with other important things to feel it.

In one of our last conversations, Alan shared with me an odd and funny teaching about death. This teaching involved his fountain pen collection, which was extensive and worth a lot of money. He had sold several thousand dollars' worth of pens to a man he'd contacted online. Before payment was mailed, the man, some years younger than Alan, suddenly died. Since there was no good record of the transaction, the attorney who was handling the estate for the widow said he would not pay. Alan could have hired his own attorney to recover the money, but it wasn't worth the trouble and expense, so he ate the loss. "But I didn't mind," he said, "because I learned something that I should have known and thought I knew but actually I didn't know: when you're dead you can't do anything." He told me this with great earnestness. As if it had never actually occurred to him that when you're dead you can't do anything.

In a memorial retreat we held a few days after Alan's death, I repeated this story. I said that since Alan was now dead and couldn't do anything anymore, we would now have to do something because we were still alive. What that something was, I didn't know. I only knew that somehow, in the face of a great loss, one does something different than one would otherwise have done.

So this is what I learned (with Alan's help) about the meaning of loss: that love rushes into the absence that is loss, and that that love brings inspired action. If we are able to give ourselves to the loss, to move toward it rather than away in an effort to escape or deny or distract or obscure, our wounded hearts become full, and out of that fullness we will do things differently and we will do different things.

The Tibetan Buddhist master Chögyam Trungpa talks about a soft spot, a raw spot, a wounded spot on the body or in the heart. A spot that is painful and sore. We hate such spots, so we try to prevent them. And if we can't prevent them, we try to cover them up so we won't absent-mindedly rub them or pour hot or cold water on them. A sore spot is no fun, but it is valuable. In *Training the Mind*, Trungpa calls the sore spot *embryonic compassion, potential compassion*. Our loss, our wound, is precious to us because it can wake us up to love, and to loving action.

Our first response to loss, difficulty, or pain is not to want to surrender to what has happened to us. It seems so negative, so wrong, and we don't want to give in to it. Yet we can't help thinking and feeling differently, and it is the thinking and the feeling, so unpleasant and painful, that is the real cause of our suffering.

When sudden loss or trouble occurs, we feel shock and bewilderment, as I did when Alan died. For so long we expected things to be as they had been, had taken this as much for granted as the air we breathe, and suddenly it is not so. Maybe tomorrow we will wake up to discover it was all just a temporary mistake and that things are back to normal. (After Alan's death I had dreams that he hadn't actually died, that it had all been some sort of correctable slip-up.)

After the shock passes, fear and despair arrive. We are anxious about our uncertain future, over which we have so little control. It is easy to fall into the paralysis of despair, caroming back to our childish default position of feeling completely vulnerable and unprepared in a harsh and hostile world. This fearful feeling of self-diminishment may darken our view to such an extent that we find ourselves wondering whether we are worthwhile people, whether we are capable of surviving in this tough world, whether we deserve to survive, whether our lives matter, whether there is any point in trying to do anything at all.

This is what it feels like when the raw spot is rubbed. The sense of loss, the despair, the fear—it is terrible and we hate it, but it is exactly what we need. It is the embryo of compassion stirring to be born. Birth is painful.

All too many people in times like these just don't have the heart to do spiritual practice. But these are the best times for practice because motivation is so clear. Practice can no longer be perceived as an option or a refinement, but only as a matter of survival. The tremendous benefit of simple meditation practice is most salient in these moments. Having exhausted all avenues of activity that might change your outward circumstances, and given up on other means of finding inner relief for your raging or sinking mind, there is nothing left to do except sit down on your chair or cushion and just be present with your situation. There you sit, feeling your body. You try to sit up straight, with some basic human dignity. You notice you are breathing. You also notice that troubling thoughts and feelings are present in the mind. You are not here to make them go away or to cover them up with pleasant and encouraging spiritual slogans. There they are, all your demons, your repetitive negative themes. Your mind is (to borrow a phrase from the poet Michael Palmer) a "museum of negativity." And you are sitting there quietly breathing inside that museum. There is nothing else to do. You can't fix anything—the situation is beyond that. Gradually it dawns on you that these dark thoughts and anxious feelings are just that—thinking, feeling. They are exhibits in the museum of negativity, but not necessarily realities of the outside world. This simple insight—that thoughts and feelings are thoughts and feelings—is slight, but it makes all the difference. You continue to sit, continue to pay attention to body and breath, and you label everything else: "thinking, thinking; feeling, feeling." Eventually, you are able to pick up your coat from the coat-check and walk out of the museum into the sunlight.

Confronting, accepting, being with negative thinking and feeling, knowing that they are not the whole of reality and not you, is the most fruitful and beneficial of all spiritual practices—better even than experiencing bliss or Oneness. You can practice it on the meditation cushion in the simple way I have described, but you can also practice it in other ways.

Journaling practice can be a big help. Keep a small notebook handy during the day and jot down an arresting word or phrase when you read or hear one. From time to time look at these words or phrases (they need not be uplifting or even sensible, they can be quite odd or random) and select the ones that attract you. These become your list of journaling prompts. When you have time, sit down with your notebook (doing this in a disciplined way, at a certain time each day, is best), choose a prompt, and write rapidly and spontaneously for ten to fifteen minutes, pen never leaving the paper, whatever comes to mind, no matter how nonsensical or irrelevant it may seem. In this way you empty out your swirling mind. You curate your own exhibition of negativity. It can be quite entertaining and even instructive.

Another way to reorient yourself with your thoughts and feelings is to share them with others. If you are feeling fear or despair, you can be sure that you are not alone. No doubt many of your friends and family members are feeling this as well. Rather than ignoring your anxieties (which tend to proliferate like mushrooms in the dark room of your closeted mind) or complaining obsessively about them to everyone you meet (which also increases the misery), you can undertake the spiritual discipline of speaking to others. Taking a topic or a prompt from your notebook, cueing off something you've read or written, or simply distilling what you have been thinking or feeling into a coherent thought can allow you to speak to one or more people in a more structured, and possibly comfortable, way.

Bring a few friends together. Divide yourselves into groups of three or four. After five minutes of silence to collect your thoughts, have each person speak as spontaneously as possible for five to seven minutes by the clock on the chosen topic. The others just listen: no questions, no comments. If it seems useful, one person can give feedback to the speaker. Not giving advice (it is a much better practice if advice and commentary is entirely outlawed) but simply reviewing for the speaker, in your own words, what you have heard him or her say. Listening to what you have said repeated back to you in another's voice can be extremely illuminating. And forgetting about your own troubles long enough to actually listen to another is a great relief. It is likely to bring out sympathy, even love. There is no better medicine than thinking of others, even if for only five minutes.

Working with these practices, you'll get a grip on the kinds of thinking and feeling that arise when conditions are difficult. The goal is not to make the thoughts and feelings go away. When there is loss or trouble it is normal to feel sorrow, fear, despair, confusion, discouragement. These feelings connect us to others who feel them as we do, so we don't want to eliminate them. But it can be good to have some perspective (and occasional relief) so these thoughts don't get the best of us and become full-blown demons pushing us around.

Back now to the basic meditation practice: when you sit, noticing the breath and the body on the chair or cushion, noticing the thoughts and feelings in the mind and heart and perhaps also the sounds in the room and the stillness, something else also begins to come into view. You notice the most fundamental of all facts: you are alive. You are a living, breathing, embodied, human being. You can actually feel this—the feeling of being alive. You can rest in this basic feeling, the nature of life, of consciousness, the underlying basis of everything you will ever experience—even the negativity. Sitting there with this basic feeling of being alive, you might begin to feel gratitude. After all, you didn't ask for this, you didn't earn it. It is just there, a gift to you. It won't last forever, but for now, in this moment, here it is, perfect, complete, and you are sharing it with everything else that exists in this stark, basic, and beautiful way. Whatever your problems and challenges may be, you are, you exist in this bright world with others, with trees, sky, water, stars, sun, and moon. If you sit there long enough and regularly enough, you will feel this, even in your darkest moments.

Based on this experience, you might reflect differently on your life. What is really important? How much do our expectations and social constructs really matter? What really counts? What is the bottom line for a human life? To be alive. Well, you are alive. To love others and be loved by others. Well, you do love, and it is within your power to love more deeply, and if you do, it is guaranteed that others will respond with more love. To be kind to others and to receive kindness is also within your power, regardless of expectations, losses, or circumstances. You need to eat every day, it is true. You need a good place to sleep at night, you need some sort of work to do, but probably you have these things, and if you do you can offer them to others. Once you overcome the sting and virulence of your naturally arising negativity and return to the feeling of being alive, you will think more clearly about what matters more and what matters less about your life, and you will see that regardless of your conditions you can participate in what matters most. You will see that you actually do have what you need, actually can feel grateful for what you already have, and actually do have plenty to do based on this gratitude.

Love After Love

Derek Walcott

The time will come
when, with elation,
you will greet yourself arriving
at your own door, in your own mirror,
and each will smile at the other's welcome,

and say, sit here. Eat.
You will love again the stranger who was your self.
Give wine. Give bread. Give back your heart
to itself, to the stranger who has loved you

all your life, whom you ignored
for another, who knows you by heart.
Take down the love letters from the bookshelf,

the photographs, the desperate notes,
peel your own image from the mirror.
Sit. Feast on your life.

A Good Enough Death

14

Joshua Bright

For more than a year, I visited and photographed a dying man named John R. Hawkins. He was being ushered from this life by a good friend, Robert Chodo Campbell, whom he had known for twenty-three years and who is a Zen priest and cofounder of the Zen Center for Contemplative Care. Their exchanges, even in the face of death and the inevitable fears that precede it, were honest and loving. John was a kind and intelligent man. During the moments he was lucid we often laughed. Other times he cried, reflecting on the past. Despite his physical deterioration, the atmosphere around John's bedside seemed to grow warmer and

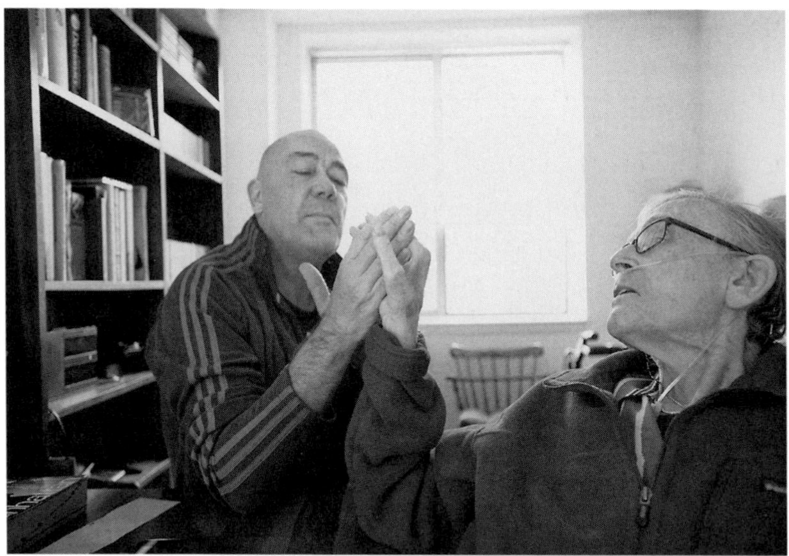

more intimate with each visit. My own uncomfortable emotions toward death began to dissipate.

I had never looked closely for a long period at a dying person. I had never listened to the strained breathing of a body barely functioning

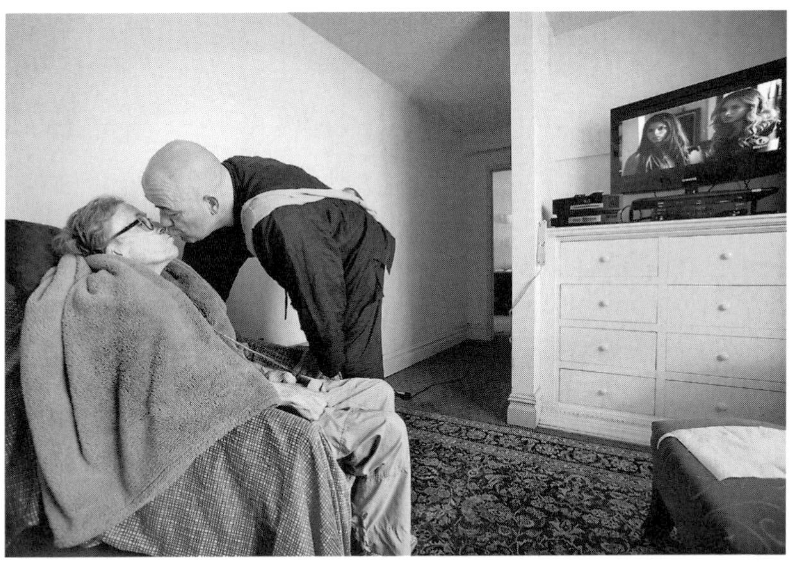

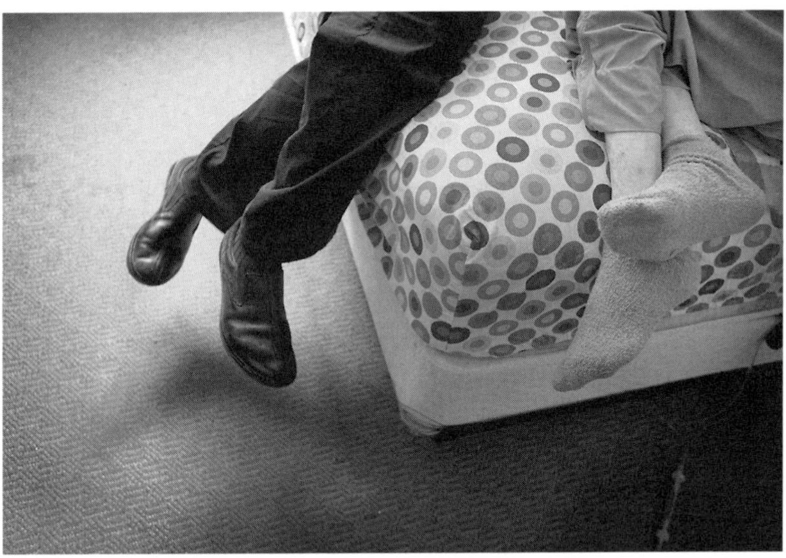

and had never put my head beside a man too weak to speak, smelled his pungent breath, and silently shared his day in, day out view of the white popcorn ceiling. Only once I put the camera down and became present did I begin to feel my fears slowly melting away.

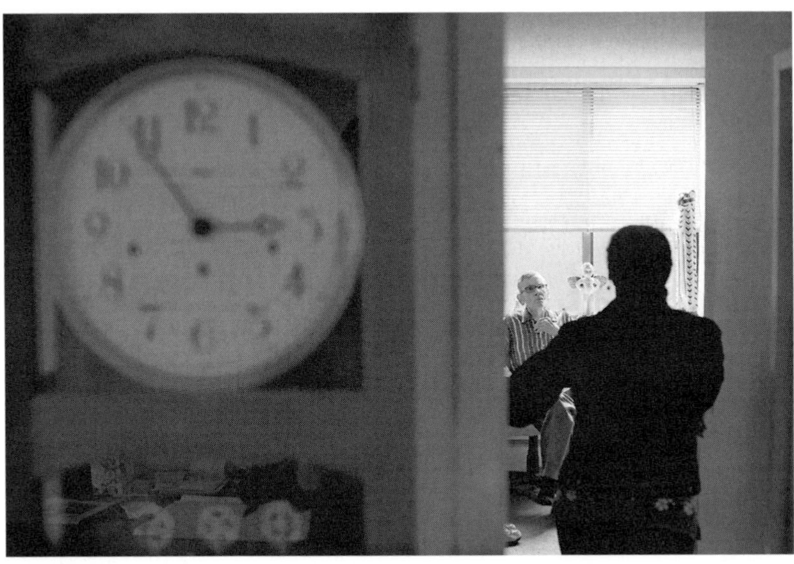

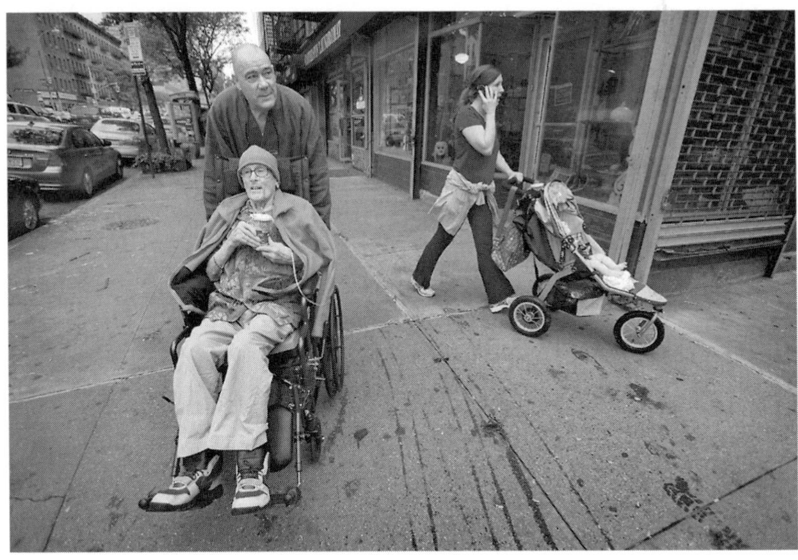

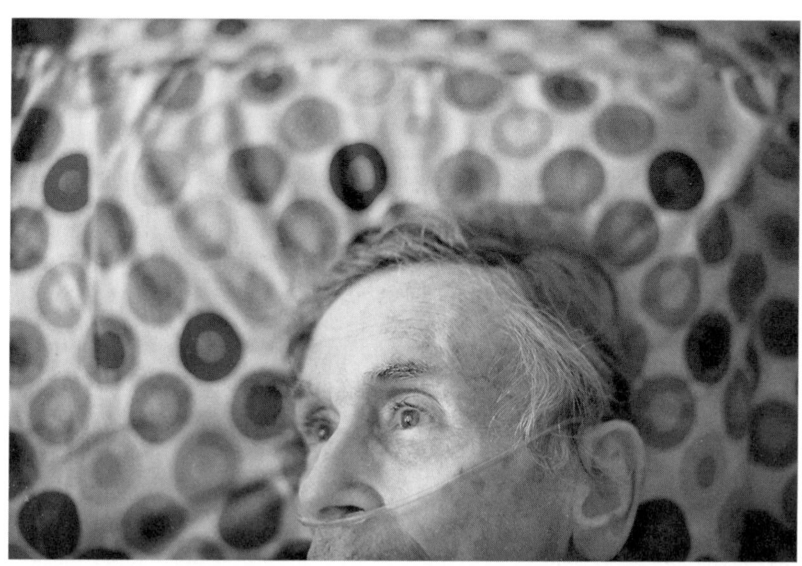

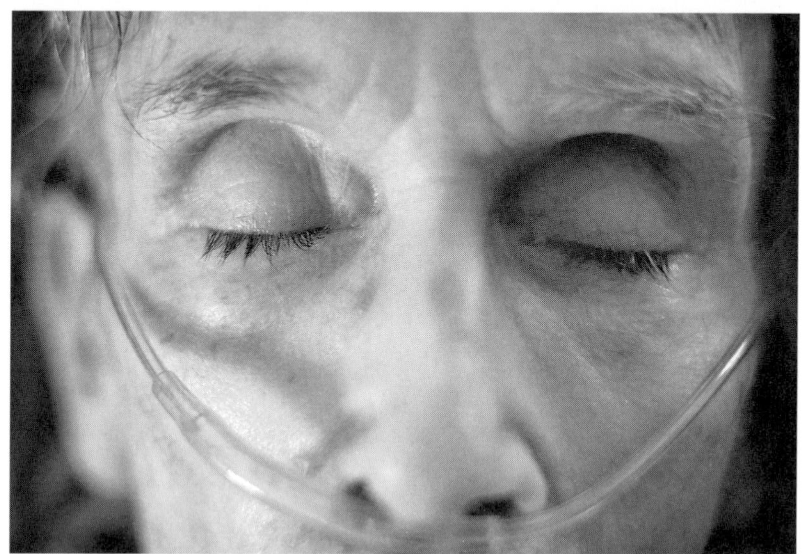

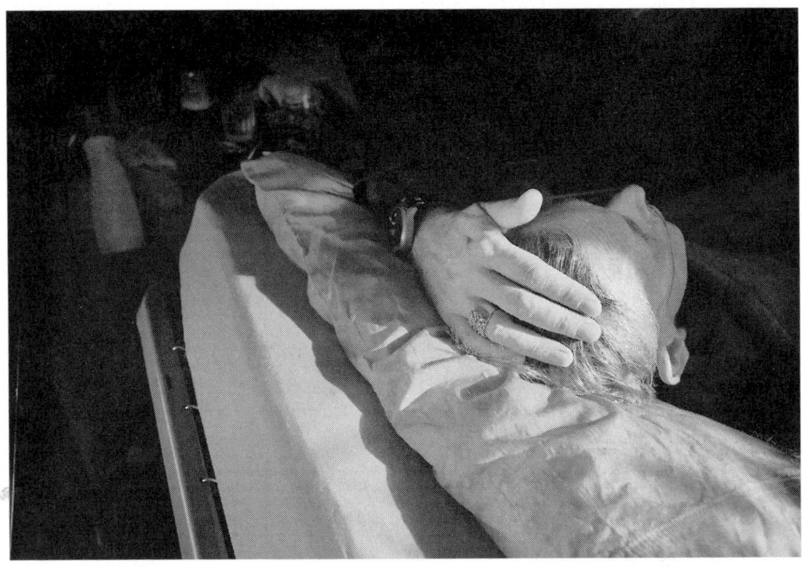

This nearness to death's physical attributes allowed me to contemplate my parents' current and serious health concerns, as well as my own mortality. My consciousness became richer for it. After leaving John's bedside to return to my wife and son, I would often feel positively euphoric, as though walking away from a therapist's office or standing on a cliff.

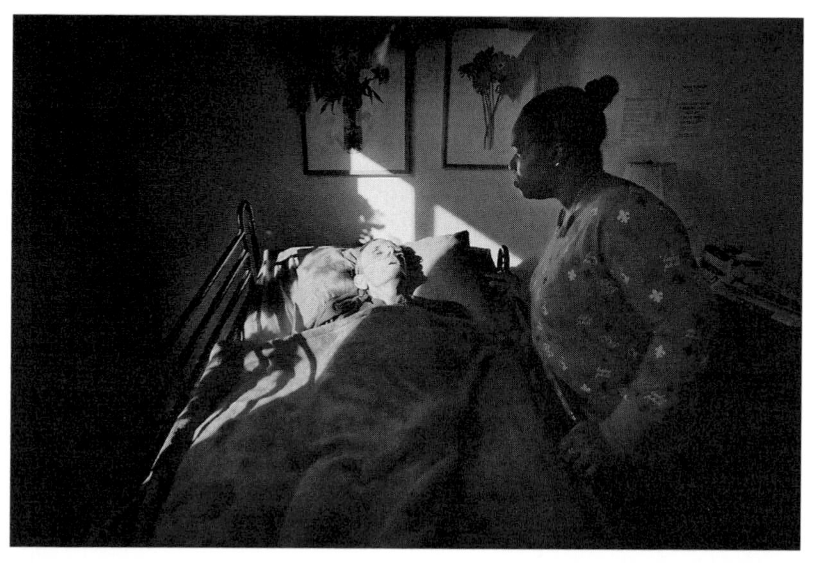

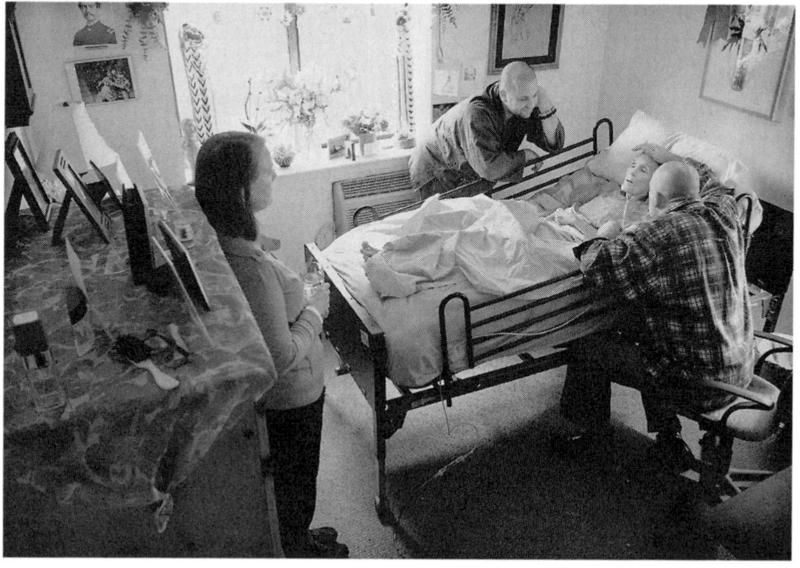

In the few hours after he died, before the people from the funeral home came, we stood around him, quietly observing the changes to his body. We saw the sinking of cheeks and eyes and the revealing of the neck bones. We felt his forehead, still warm even after his limbs had grown cold. We talked about death and I took some photos and we teased the man who was now gone and we laughed. Gradually, his mouth pulled itself into the cheeky smile we all knew so well.

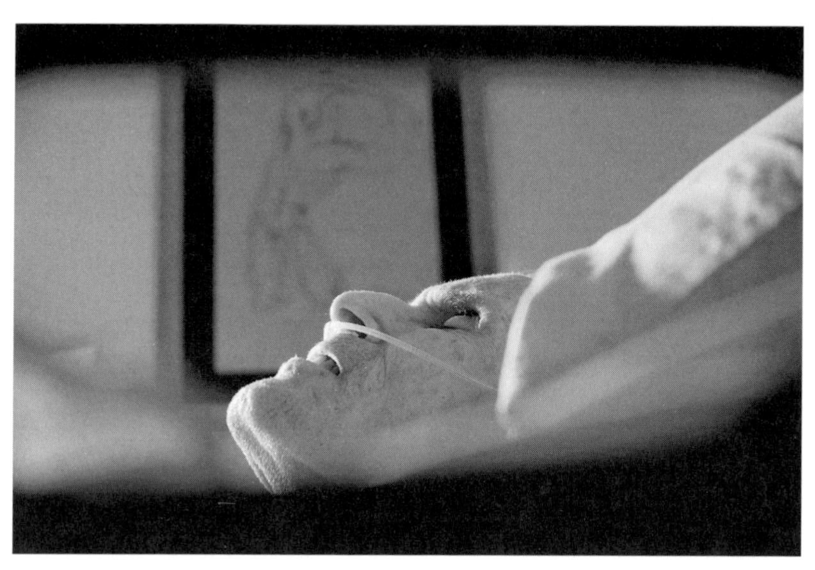

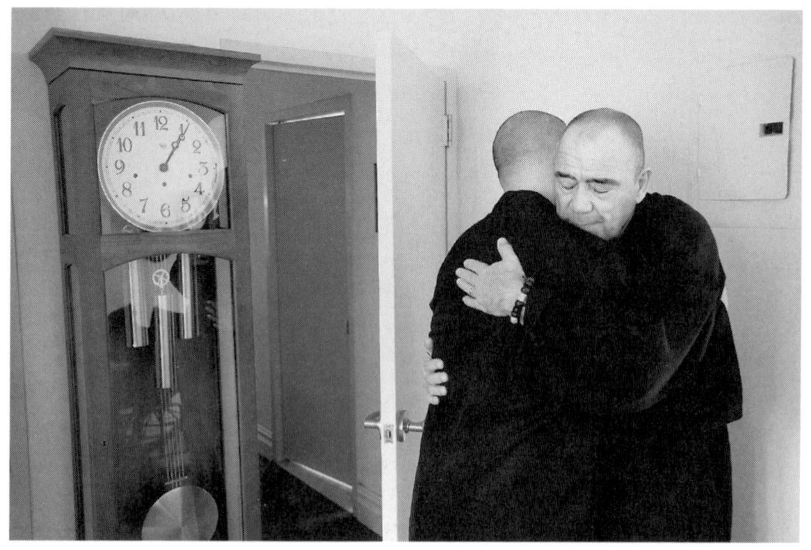

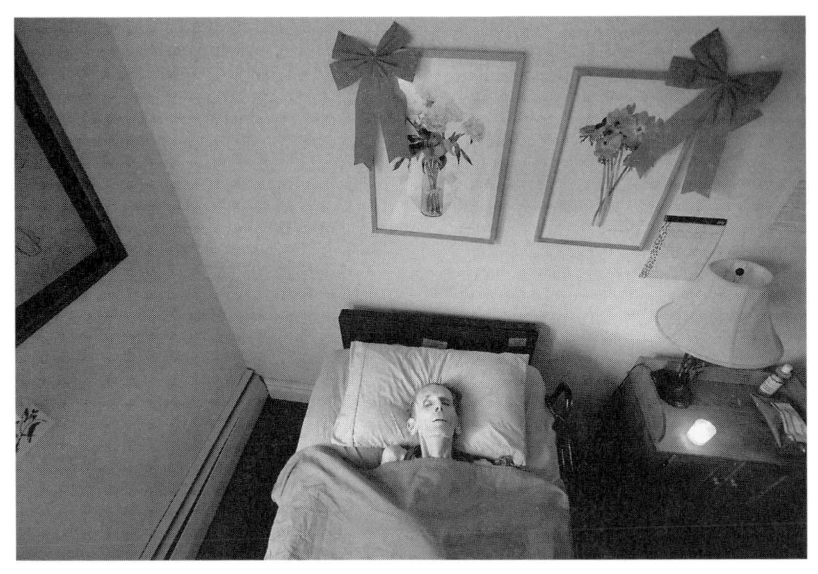

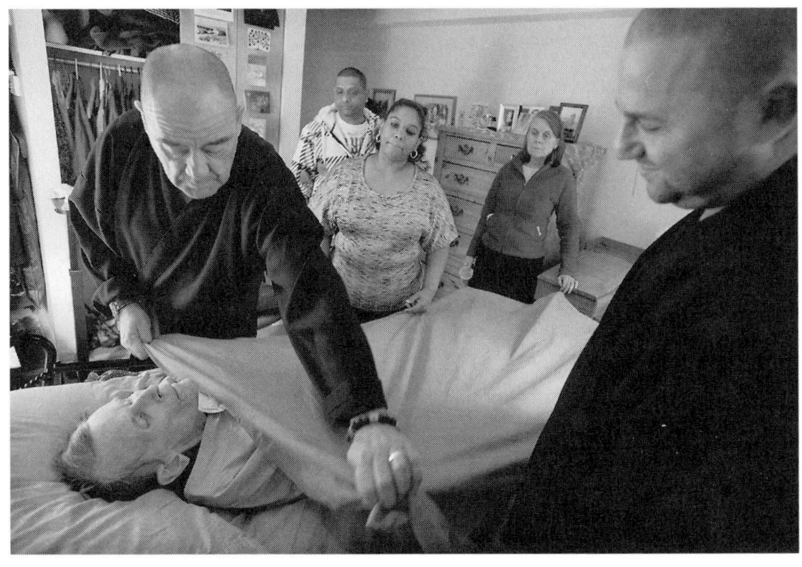

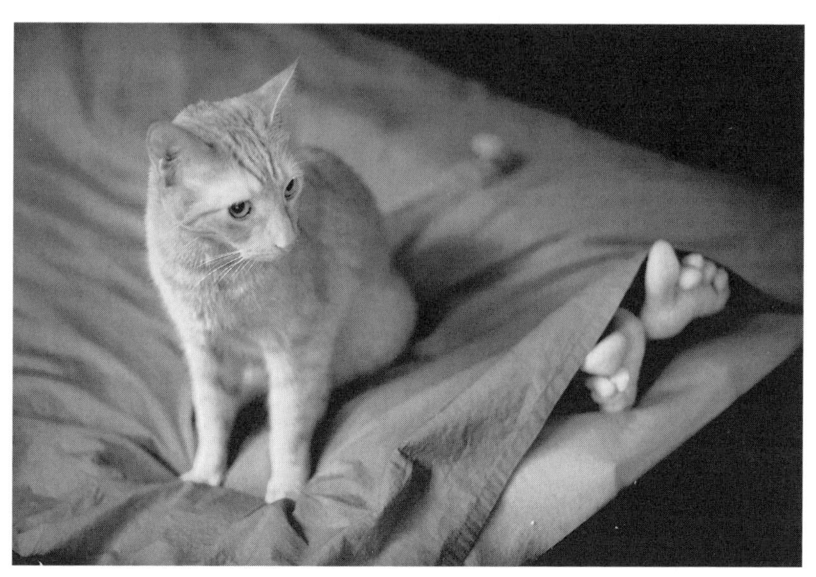

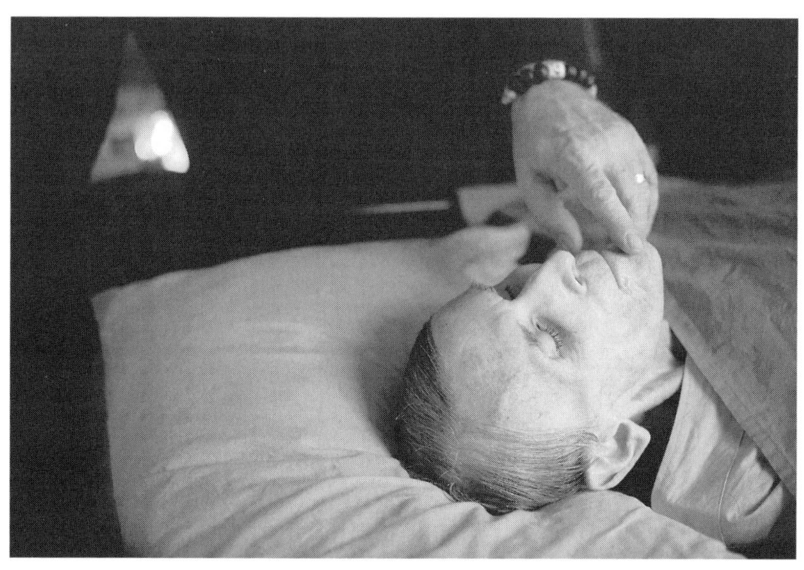

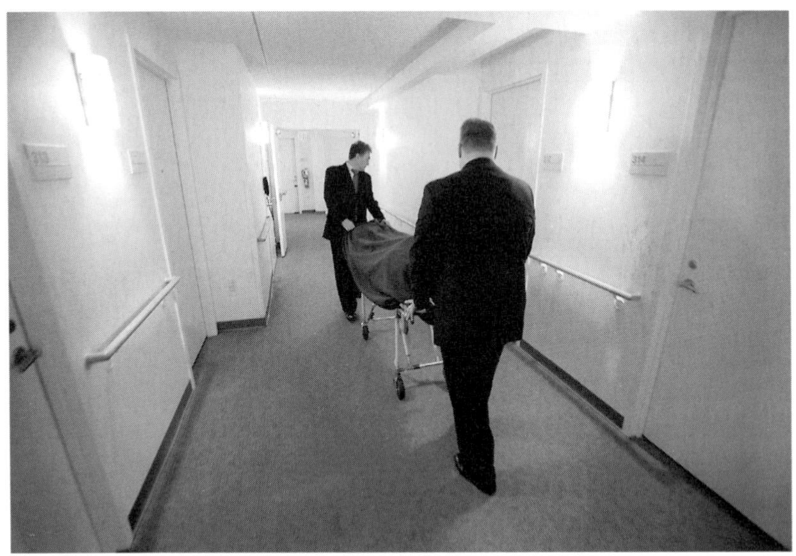

We could use news of a good enough death. Not a tragic death or a famous death, just a good enough one. The kind that might happen to any of us, if we are present.

A Theravada Approach to Spiritual Care of the Dying and Deceased

15

Gil Fronsdal

Death and dying have central roles in most traditions. They are important catalysts for engaging in practice and frequently used as themes of reflection. In offering spiritual care one should be prepared to respond to people's needs and concerns related to death. For example, monastics, teachers, and caregivers may be called on to discuss existential issues related to our mortality, offer instructions in practices related to death, counsel and guide the dying, and offer support to family and friends of the dying or the dead. In addition, an important role for spiritual caregivers may be to officiate funerals and memorial services.

What follows are some general notes on a Theravadan perspective on some of these issues.

While different Buddhist traditions have varied customs around dying and death, an enduring understanding in all these traditions is that death is not a final end. For people who are not fully enlightened, rebirth follows death. Regarding those individuals who are fully awakened, it is considered impossible to make any assertion about what happens after death, including the idea that they are or are not reborn. However, even though Buddhist traditions share in the idea of rebirth, there are differences among some of the traditions in how they understand the various destinations and forms of rebirth a person might take. There are also differences within traditions (and between Buddhist teachers) how much emphasis or importance is put on the notion of rebirth. For some, the emphasis is on practicing fully in this life without any thought for what will follow. For others, planning for and arranging for favorable rebirths is the central thrust of their religious practice.

The notion of rebirth brings much solace to those who are distressed by the alternative. However, there are many people for whom the idea of rebirth is itself distressing as they imagine some of the unfortunate circumstances they are headed for. In classic Indian Buddhism, being stuck in an endless cycle of birth, death, and rebirth is considered undesirable, and the ultimate direction of Buddhist practice is to be released from this cycle. It is understood that the fuel for further rebirth is clinging, and once this fuel has been fully dissolved, death will not lead to further rebirth.

Whether one believes in the literal idea of rebirth or not, all Buddhists understand that clinging also fuels the constant cycle of suffering that is born and dies in our minds each unliberated moment. The work of waking up and becoming free of these momentary cycles is the same work of becoming free from the cycles of rebirth. People who believe in rebirth sometimes have the advantage of having greater motivation for spiritual practice than those who focus only on freedom within this lifetime.

Whether one believes in rebirth or not, dying is a time when we are confronted with life's deepest truths. To be able to learn and be transformed by these truths is one of the ultimate tasks of Buddhist practice.

Preparing for Death

In all circumstances connected to death and dying, the most important offering of the caregiver is his or her own equanimity and lack of conflict regarding death. Engaging in reflections and practices that prepare one for death is perhaps the most important preparation the caregiver needs to do to be ready to respond wisely and compassionately to people facing issues of death and dying. An important role of caregivers is to encourage people to consider the reality of death. To do this with authenticity and credibility, the caregiver needs to have done this for herself or himself.

Theravada Buddhism encourages people to prepare for death. This preparation is considered part of living a mindful, conscientious life, as preparing helps make the circumstance of dying easier for everyone concerned. There are both practical and spiritual aspects to such readiness. To have our affairs in order simplifies our own life when death approaches, and so it is easier to focus on what is most important at that time. It is also an expression of goodwill for our family and friends since it simplifies their work in caring for us and our possessions both before and after our death. To be spiritually and emotionally prepared for our death optimizes the chances that we can use the period of dying for its unparalleled opportunity for Buddhist practice. When appropriate, caregivers should encourage people to be prepared for their death.

In a sense, all Buddhist practice prepares a person to die. For example, people who meditate regularly will generally have less fear of death than people who don't; they will have developed some of the inner qualities that help bring balance and equanimity in the face of death. With the development of concentration, for instance, the mind tends to remain more balanced and less reactive than a mind without this stabilizing force. With the development of mindfulness, meditators have a deep appreciation of moment-to-moment impermanence—the birth and death that happen every instant. This can also provide the trust or confidence to go along with the letting-go process of dying. Because it helps us to be present for what is happening without being caught by aversion, desire, or doubt, the best single preparation for death is mindfulness meditation. Also, the insights of mindfulness practice are the springboards to liberation. The ability to practice mindfulness on one's deathbed is considered one of the most opportune times for liberation.

In addition, Buddhism encourages people to take the time to actually contemplate the topic of death. In Theravada Buddhism, meditators are encouraged to practice reflecting on the "four protections," which are said to support the deepening of meditation practice. These four are the contemplation of the qualities of the Buddha to protect us from doubt and discouragement, the practice of loving-kindness for anger, contemplating the unappetizing aspects of the body to calm desire (especially sexual desire), and the contemplation of death as a protection from heedlessness and laziness. Instead of avoiding the topic, one is encouraged to confront it as directly as possible and to recognize that death is inherent in life. Some teachers instruct practitioners to maintain death as a constant companion. One way to do this is to wear a *mala*, or string of Buddhist prayer beads, made of bone, each bead sculpted in the shape of a skull.

Contemplation of death can also help keep one's priorities straight, and it can be a catalyst for getting serious about one's spiritual practice. In fact, the great Tibetan yogi Milarepa said, "Without mindfulness of death, whatever Dharma practice you take up will be merely superficial." Confronting death directly also allows us to work through our fear, aversion, and confusion around death. Done well, the contemplation of death can help bring a deep sense of peace and well-being.

In the discourses of the Buddha, the contemplation of death is integrated with the overall development of mindfulness. The sutta on the Four Foundations of Mindfulness lists nine different contemplations on a corpse at different stages of decay. One is to remind oneself that as this corpse has the nature to decay, so one's own body has the nature to decay as well. Since nowadays bodies are not allowed to decay in charnel grounds, some people have adapted this practice to one of visiting hospitals or morgues where one might have permission to sit with a corpse. Sometimes people will have a photo of a dead person and use that as a focus of this contemplation.

One of the best resources for practicing the contemplation on death is Larry Rosenberg's book *Living in the Light of Death*. He offers the following death awareness practices:

1. Awareness of the inevitability of death
   - A. Reflecting that everyone must die
   - B. Reflecting that our life span is decreasing continuously
   - C. Reflecting that the time for developing our minds is small

2. Awareness of the time of death
   D. Reflecting that human life expectancy is uncertain
   E. Reflecting that there are many causes of death
   F. Reflecting that the human body is so fragile
3. Awareness that only insight into Dharma can help us at the time of death
   G. Reflecting that our possessions and enjoyments cannot help
   H. Reflecting that our loved ones cannot help
   I. Reflecting that our own body cannot help

Rosenberg recommends practicing these reflections for about twenty minutes a day after first calming the mind—through breath meditation, for example. Each day one focuses on one of the reflections. Sometimes the practice can simply entail repeating one of the contemplations and then exploring the feelings, thoughts, and body sensations that arise. For example, one could say to oneself, "Everyone must die." In addition one can actively think or contemplate each phrase and its meanings, implications, and value.

The various mindfulness practices around death are not meant to be morbid or distressing contemplations. In fact, if that is the result, one should probably not bother with the practices or should talk to a teacher about one's experience.

While these practices have been Buddhist meditations since ancient times, they are perhaps particularly important in our modern times where death and dying usually happen privately, beyond the view of regular daily life. Buddhism encourages us to see death as a natural occurrence.

Being prepared to die also entails healing any relationships with conflict or unfinished business. Hopefully, such relationships are dealt with as soon as possible, well before an impending death. Since death can arrive unexpectedly, it is important not to delay resolving our difficulties with others. Buddhist resources for this work include loving-kindness and forgiveness practices, confession and apologies where needed, and the practices of honesty, ethics, and generosity. Even if the other party in a conflict does not want reconciliation, it is still possible to do the inner work of releasing one's own resentment, anger, or fear. It is hard to die peacefully if we die with resentments or regrets.

Easing the Dying Process

It can be extremely difficult to really understand and accept the fact that one is dying. One might remain in denial about how serious the situation is. Or one may hold on to hope at all costs. Or someone might be seriously sick, but there remains real medical hope for recovery even right up to the time of death. The advantage of fully accepting one's approaching death is that it gives the person the opportunity to live accordingly. When appropriate, it can be the role of the caregiver or teacher to help dying people to wisely "turn the corner."

When a Buddhist practitioner knows he or she is going to die, their practice becomes extremely important. In fact, when death is inevitable, one would hopefully put aside as much time as possible for practice. Some people find it important to have lots of support for practice. They might invite friends or sangha members to their home or hospital room to meditate with them. They might arrange for regular interviews with a Buddhist teacher to discuss their practice and concerns. Other people prefer having lots of solitude and silence as they die. If, for whatever reason, you do not have the ability to maintain your own practice, ask friends or teachers to lead you in guided meditation or to read passages of spiritual wisdom or instruction.

The nature of one's spiritual practice will change depending on where one is in the dying process. At times, practice may be quite active and directed, for example in healing interpersonal issues, cultivating loving-kindness and forgiveness, and developing one's concentration and calm. At other times, the practice may mostly entail deeper and deeper forms of letting go and surrender. When one experiences fear, anger, or other painful emotions, these too should be seen as important parts of the overall dying process to be included in one's mindfulness practice.

The goal in dying is to try to die with as much awareness as possible and in a wholesome state of mind. Mindfulness itself is a wholesome activity of mind, and so some people simply focus on continuing with the mindfulness practice as long as they can. One of the reasons for healing interpersonal relationships is to mitigate being plagued by unpleasant feelings while one is dying. A number of practices are recommended for improving the quality of one's mind. For example, one can recall one's good deeds, virtues, or memories. One can think about the Buddha or other inspiring spiritual teachers. One can practice loving-kindness to gladden the mind. One can perform acts of generosity. One can arrange for one's environment to be as peaceful and spiritually supportive as possible. Some people set up an altar or have pictures of loved ones or important spiritual teachers placed around the room.

How to Care for the Dying

It is easy for caregivers to focus exclusively on the needs of the person dying. However, in order to offer the best spiritual care, it is important that the caregivers be self-aware enough to be able to monitor the state of their own mind. If we want to help a person die with as much peace, acceptance, and love as possible, the caregiver needs to aim toward having these qualities established in him- or herself. This does not mean that these qualities need to be present; it means that we take responsibility for how we are feeling. Caregivers themselves may need support, and it's important to search it out. Caring for the dying can be a spiritual practice in its own right that can support the spiritual practice of the dying.

The caregiver also needs to be sensitive to the family, friends, and caregivers around the dying. When family and friends can't let go of the dying person, it can be harder for the person to die. Sometimes it can be wise for the caregiver to help family and friends to resolve their clingings. If this involves resentment or a grudge toward the dying person, the caregiver may encourage a process of forgiveness. Close to the time of death it may be helpful for family and friends to indicate that as much as they love the person, it is okay for the person to die and that they will be okay after the person has died. If appropriate, the caregiver should try to help the family and friends to grant the dying person permission to die.

The time shortly before death is extremely important and requires attending caregivers to use their best judgment and intuition as to what is needed. If the dying person can speak, it is of course easy to know their wishes. If he or she can't speak but has previously given instructions for what to do, then also it might be relatively easy to know what to do. If the person is not speaking and has left no instructions, then one must intuit what is needed. Whatever one does, it is best to softly tell the person before doing so. Even if a person is unconscious or in a coma, it is best to assume that the person can hear you and to tell the person what you think the person needs to hear.

Whenever possible, a caregiver should try to find out in advance the answers to the following questions:

- Where does the person want to die?
- Who, if anyone, does the person want to be present at the time of death? Who does the person want to be notified as their death approaches?
- What does the person want while dying or when dead (specific practices, rituals, readings, chants, music, guided meditations, people in meditation in the room)? This can include instruction concerning what to do with one's body, and desires for the memorial service.

It's important that the environment around the dying person be peaceful. Often this can best be accomplished at home. If a person is going to die in a hospital then effort should be made to have the hospital room peaceful. Perhaps an altar can be set up, flowers displayed, and pictures put on the wall.

We cannot always know when the final moment of death has occurred. Sometimes it's assumed that death occurs when the breath stops. However, there is a belief in Theravada Buddhism that death is final when the breath stops *and* the body has become cold. This means that the process of letting go may continue for a while after the breath stops. Sometimes people sense the consciousness or life force leaving the body, and this is recognized as the moment of death.

Sometimes there can be a sense that the person's consciousness hovers for some time in the room. Generally the final moment or moments of death are peaceful, and the peacefulness of it can be quite palpable. During this peaceful period immediately after the last breath, it is best to assume that the person can still hear what is being said. If it seems appropriate, one can softly speak to the person. One might continue giving the person instructions in letting go, read sacred texts, practice loving-kindness toward the person, chant the refuge chant, or meditate in the stillness. During this intermediate period after the breath has stopped, it is recommended that the body not be touched in case such contact may disturb or confuse the letting go process of dying. While someone's death may trigger great grief, it is recommended that the room where someone has died remain as quiet and peaceful as possible. If possible, loud expressions of grief should be reserved for later or be done elsewhere. The reason for this is so that the expressions of grief do not confuse or affect the person who is dying/has died.

Keeping the Body after Death

After a person has died, the body should be treated with respect, honoring the memory of the person. In the case of a sudden, unexpected death, the body will probably have to go to the coroner for an autopsy. There are no Theravada religious teachings that object to an autopsy. If a person dies in a hospital, the hospital may have limitations on how long the body can remain in a hospital room. If a person dies at home, a doctor or the coroner must be contacted so a death certificate can be issued. But once a person has died, there is no need to immediately contact anyone. Even if someone dies in a hospital room, you can wait some time before you inform the staff. In all circumstances, make contact with a nurse, doctor, or coroner when you are ready. If a person dies at home and you are told to call 911, be prepared that emergency medics might come rushing to your house. Efforts should be made to head them off at the front door so that they don't unnecessarily disturb the atmosphere in the house.

In the Theravada tradition, once a person has died there is no particular practice or teaching about leaving the body undisturbed for any period of time. Sometimes burial or cremation happens as quickly as possible, and sometimes the body is kept at home for several days. Sometimes there can be an actual or ritual washing of the body. Giving friends and family a chance to sit with the dead body can help their grieving process. People who don't have this opportunity will sometimes have a harder time accepting that the person is really dead. Leaving the body at home for a day or more can help maintain a reverent, perhaps sacred atmosphere to mark a person's death. If this is desired, there is the option of inviting in sangha members to sit and chant with the body. If a person dies in a hospital or away from home, it is sometimes possible to bring the body home, unless an autopsy is needed. If it adds to the distress of family and friends to keep the body for more than a short while, there is no problem in having a mortuary service come for the body.

In some of the Mahayana Buddhist traditions, there is the practice of leaving the body alone for some time after death as a way of helping the departed through the intermediate state before the next rebirth. While the intermediate state can last up to forty-nine days, a common custom is to leave the body undisturbed for three days. During this time, people can come to meditate in the room with the body, perform Buddhist ceremonies such as the refuge ceremony, or continue to give instructions to the departed to help them negotiate the intermediate state.

While Theravada Buddhism does not hold the view of an extended intermediate period, there is sometimes a belief that the deceased person in his or her next rebirth can still benefit from things done for them. This means that while the beliefs are different, the practice of helping the departed is shared by both traditions. Theravada practices done for the departed are usually acts of merit. This can include doing a refuge ceremony, chanting Buddhist teachings, practicing acts of generosity in the name of the deceased, or dedicating merit to the departed. It is believed that these meritorious acts can benefit the departed if he or she is aware of the acts and rejoices in them.

If a caregiver arrives after the person has died, he or she should discern what role is expected. Often the family and friends will look to the caregiver for guidance, especially in terms of spiritual and ritual matters. Generally it is good to immediately sit down next to the body of the departed and meditate with eyes open, taking in whatever presence of the person might still remain in the room. Even if no presence can be "felt," practicing mindfulness while being open or "receptive" to the possibility can be helpful. Alternatively, or in addition, the caregiver can focus mindfulness on whatever stillness or peace can be sensed in the room. After a short time of doing this, the caregiver can do any of the things mentioned above for when a person is dying or just passed away.

Funerals, Cremations, Memorial Services, and Rites of Transition

Funerals, cremation rituals, and memorial services can be conducted in a great variety of ways that fulfill the wishes and needs of the departed and/or meet the needs and sensibilities of those participating in the service. There is no fixed Theravada way of conducting these services. In Theravada countries and in South East Asian communities in the US, it is customary to have services officiated by monks. Caregivers or teachers in America who are asked to conduct memorial or funeral services are rarely expected to perform predominantly ritual-centered services (expect perhaps for burials). Most Vipassana teachers will design a service around the desires of the departed, if known, and in consultation with close family members.

The two primary functions for these services are to help the departed and to help the living. In helping the departed, the rituals function as a rite of transition, helping the person move on to his or her next life. In general, funerals and cremations are likely to have a stronger "rite of transition" aspect than memorials.

In helping the living, these services are ways of helping people process the loss of a relative, friend, colleague, neighbor, etc. Some people appreciate the chance to express the range of feelings they might have, including anger. Other people find it most helpful if the service focuses on celebrating the departed's life, perhaps recalling how the person enriched the lives of others.

What follows is a general outline with the most common elements I use when officiating a memorial service. They are listed in the order that they might occur during a service. In designing a ceremony, the different elements can be used and ordered as appropriate.

1. Opening statement: Welcomes everyone, states the purpose and perhaps the intention of the service. Attempts to set the appropriate mood, e.g. celebratory, subdued, reverent, irreverent, religious, secular, formal, informal.
2. Chanting: This would include the core Theravada chants either in English or in Pali: Homage to the Buddha (Namo tassa . . .), The Three Refuges, Taking the Five Precepts, and the funeral verse, which follows.

   Annicā vata saṅkhārā, Uppāda vaya dhammino.
   Uuppajjitvā nirujjhanti Tesam vūpasamo sukho.

   All things are impermanent; they arise and pass away.
   Having arisen, they come to an end; their coming to
   peace is bliss.

   These chants can be done in the name of the departed, as if done in proxy. If an altar is set up with a picture of the departed or with his or her ashes, the caregiver should face the altar as though the person is there.

3. Speaking to the departed: Here the caregiver speaks directly to the departed telling them what they need to hear or encouraging them in some way. Many of the things said to a person as they die or right after death can be said here. The caregiver can also use readings from Buddhist texts for this purpose. "The Flower Poem" is sometimes read here.
4. Eulogy: Given either by the caregiver or by someone else.
5. Statements from family and friends: This can be statements given by people decided on before the service or it can be impromptu. Whoever wants to can stand up to speak. If the caregiver has addressed the departed earlier in the service, the family and friends can be invited to either address the departed directly or to speak to those assembled for the service.
6. Loving-kindness: Either a guided meditation on loving-kindness for the departed or a reading of the Metta Sutta.
7. Chanting: *"Earth returns to earth, fire returns to fire, wind returns to wind, water returns to water, space returns to space, consciousness returns to consciousness. The path of liberation plunges into peace."*
8. Closing statement.
9. Dedicating the merit of the service and of the assembled people to the welfare of the departed. And if appropriate expanding the dedication to include the welfare of all beings.

Other elements sometimes included are songs, music, poems, and slide-shows of the person's life.

Touch Me

Stanley Kunitz

Summer is late, my heart.
Words plucked out of the air
some forty years ago
when I was wild with love
and torn almost in two
scatter like leaves this night
of whistling wind and rain.
It is my heart that's late,
it is my song that's flown.
Outdoors all afternoon
under a gunmetal sky
staking my garden down,
I kneeled to the crickets trilling
underfoot as if about
to burst from their crusty shells;
and like a child again
marveled to hear so clear
and brave a music pour
from such a small machine.
What makes the engine go?
Desire, desire, desire.
The longing for the dance
stirs in the buried life.
One season only,
                                        and it's done.
So let the battered old willow

thrash against the windowpanes
and the house timbers creak.
Darling, do you remember
the man you married? Touch me,
remind me who I am.

Passing Through

Stanley Kunitz
—on my seventy-ninth birthday

Nobody in the widow's household
ever celebrated anniversaries.
In the secrecy of my room
I would not admit I cared
that my friends were given parties.
Before I left town for school
my birthday went up in smoke
in a fire at City Hall that gutted
the Department of Vital Statistics.
If it weren't for a census report
of a five-year-old White Male
sharing my mother's address
at the Green Street tenement in Worcester
I'd have no documentary proof
that I exist. You are the first,
my dear, to bully me
into these festive occasions.

Sometimes, you say, I wear
an abstracted look that drives you
up the wall, as though it signified
distress or disaffection.
Don't take it so to heart.
Maybe I enjoy not-being as much
as being who I am. Maybe

it's time for me to practice
growing old. The way I look
at it, I'm passing through a phase:
gradually I'm changing to a word.
Whatever you choose to claim
of me is always yours;
nothing is truly mine
except my name. I only
borrowed this dust.

The Layers

Stanley Kunitz

I have walked through many lives,
some of them my own,
and I am not who I was,
though some principle of being
abides, from which I struggle
not to stray.
When I look behind,
as I am compelled to look
before I can gather strength
to proceed on my journey,
I see the milestones dwindling
toward the horizon
and the slow fires trailing
from the abandoned camp-sites,
over which scavenger angels
wheel on heavy wings.
Oh, I have made myself a tribe
out of my true affections,
and my tribe is scattered!
How shall the heart be reconciled
to its feast of losses?
In a rising wind
the manic dust of my friends,
those who fell along the way,
bitterly stings my face.
Yet I turn, I turn,

exulting somewhat,
with my will intact to go
wherever I need to go,
and every stone on the road
precious to me.
In my darkest night,
when the moon was covered
and I roamed through wreckage,
a nimbus-clouded voice
directed me:
"Live in the layers,
not on the litter."
Though I lack the art
to decipher it,
no doubt the next chapter
in my book of transformations
is already written.
I am not done with my changes.

More Than Just a Medical Event 16

Kirsten DeLeo

Those who are dying have taught me three essential things: to "show up" even when I don't know what to say or do, to be myself, and to not be afraid to care. And a fourth thing, most important of all: that the moment of death is more than just a medical event.

Being with the dying is always personal—it does not matter in what role or capacity we're serving them. A dying person requires our professional skills and knowledge but, most essentially, he or she needs us to connect with them on a fundamental level, from one human being to another. And with the relentless pace and pressures in healthcare today, we can easily get caught up in how "good" a professional job we're doing, not seeing that often what the person in front of us most needs is our undistracted presence, if even for just a few moments.

I remember once teaching a group of young pediatric residents. I could feel the passion they had for their work and their love for their young patients, but I could also see their fear of being vulnerable and the pressure to bury their own emotions. One doctor admitted with disarming honesty, "It's often easier to feign compassion and interest than to show up." Another resident added, "I'm always thinking about what I have to do next, so I'm never really fully there in the moment." After a long pause, another young doctor ventured, "It's tough just to *be* when you don't know what to *say*." As many of the other group members nodded, he continued, "It's hard to allow myself to forgive and accept how I am. In the medical profession, it's common to never accept who you are, to always try to be better."

Listening to these young doctors, I was struck more strongly than ever before by the clear and urgent need for support in learning how to make the courageous and fundamental shift from *doing* to *being*. How can we keep alive the passion and joy that naturally arise through caring for our patients, while at the same time continuing to nurture the strength of heart necessary to remain present in the face of suffering?

Many years ago, I sat at the bedside of one of my very first patients—a young man, twenty-seven years old, the same age as me at the time. Cancer was consuming his body. All he wanted was to live, but it was clear that he was dying. Looking at him, it was as if I were looking into the fierce mirror of my own reality. I felt helpless and afraid. My heart was breaking. Over time, out of concern and love for my patients, I learned to "keep my seat" in those challenging moments—to simply bear witness.

My meditation practice has helped me with this; it's given me the courage to stay present with difficult emotions, mine or others, without judgment. Still, I wondered over the years if there's anything more that would help me to drop back into just being in a deeper way. How can I return to *presence* when I get caught up in my own self-concerns and fears? How can I respond to the existential and spiritual needs that surface at the threshold of life and death?

One day, with the very same questions in my heart, I found myself at a meditation center called Dzogchen Beara perched high on the clifftops overlooking the Irish sea. Sogyal Rinpoche, the Tibetan master and author of *The Tibetan Book of Living and Dying*, was leading a retreat. With an incredible sense of humor and great spaciousness, he directly addressed one of our society's greatest taboos: death. Over the years, my memory has lost the exact words he used, so I've returned again and again to his book for wisdom:

> Do we not all have a right, as we are dying, not only to have our bodies treated with respect, but also, and perhaps even

> more important, our spirits? . . . My master Dudjom Rinpoche used to say that to help a dying person is like holding out a hand to someone who is on the point of falling over, to lift them up. Through the strength and peace and deep compassionate attention of your presence, you will help them awaken their own strength. The quality of your *presence* at this most vulnerable and extreme moment is all-important.

In my search for a different way of caring, one that considers the inner dimension of life, I found a particular exercise to be tremendously supportive and transformative: an adaptation of a Tibetan Buddhist practice known as *phowa*.

Phowa is considered by Tibetan Buddhists to be the most valuable and powerful practice for the moment of death; it's meant to guide and support the transference of consciousness that occurs when a person dies. Essential Phowa, as we call our version, has become one of the core contemplative practices of this program. It creates a calm and peaceful atmosphere that benefits not only the dying person but also the caregiver, whether it be in the ICU, ER, hospice, or at home. It is a powerful reminder that death is more than just a medical event—it can be a truly sacred moment. Essential Phowa can be done by anyone; we can do it for ourselves or for others.

The beauty of the practice is that it can be adapted to an individual's own beliefs and thoughts, to what resonates and gives a sense of refuge, peace, or comfort. Neither the person offering the practice nor the person receiving it has to subscribe to the Buddhist belief system—or any belief system—for the practice to be effective. When I teach the Essential Phowa to others, a common concern is what to do if we do not know the person's personal beliefs or tradition. What if we do it *wrong*? Whether the person we practice for follows a particular religious or spiritual tradition, or none at all, we are in no way harming or disrespecting the person's beliefs and convictions.

Amazingly, Essential Phowa is not only a practice for the moment of death, but it's also a practice for healing. Some may see this as a sort of contradiction: how can a practice that helps someone die well at the same time support health? Our common dualistic mindset views life and death—living and dying—as two separate things. Consequently, we assume that we either have to put all our energy into getting better or let go of all hope and prepare to die. This either/or approach can cause tremendous anxiety when we are confronted with a potentially life-threatening illness. Hope and fear can run havoc. Am I living, or am I dying?

The practice of Essential Phowa can support the healing process of an ill person, *and* it can also support the spiritual palliation of someone who is dying. Essential Phowa is wonderfully helpful for that deeper, inner process that can take place when it is time to say goodbye, such as mending broken relationships, or discovering or reconnecting with a source of refuge or love. Moreover, this practice can also be used after someone has died as a way of offering our continued spiritual support. A number of the graduates of our program run bereavement groups, and they share Essential Phowa in their meetings. They report that the practice is a tremendous consolation to people who are grieving. It offers the bereaved something they can do for the person they have lost—a profound way of showing their love and support—which seems to lessen feelings of helplessness.

How does the practice work? If you practice for yourself, visualize in the space in front of you or above your head the embodiment of whatever truth, wisdom, and infinite love resonates with you most deeply and opens your heart. This could be a religious figure like the Buddha or Amitabha or Jesus, or perhaps a spiritual teacher. If you don't have a specific religious affiliation or don't feel you can relate to spiritual figures, don't worry. As Sogyal Rinpoche says:

> If you don't feel linked with any particular spiritual figure, simply imagine a form of pure golden light in the sky before you. The important point is that you consider the being you

> are visualizing or whose presence you feel *is* the embodiment of the truth, wisdom, and compassion of all the buddhas, saints, masters, and enlightened beings. Don't worry if you cannot visualize them very clearly. Just fill your heart with their presence and trust that they are there.

So you focus your mind, heart, and soul on the presence you have invoked. Next, you imagine that this infinitely loving, compassionate, and wise presence is deeply moved by your heartfelt and sincere wish. The presence looks at you with a loving, warm gaze and, from its heart, sends out love and compassion in the form of a stream of rays of golden light. These light rays touch all aspects of your being. Strongly feel that they reach the deepest corners of your mind and heart, the places touched by illness or where there is fear of illness. As these light rays keep streaming down to you, visualize that they heal whatever needs healing. Imagine they offer forgiveness, understanding, and peace. Imagine that they heal any past negativity, troubling history, unfinished business, destructive emotions, and pain—even including any deeper, hidden sources of your suffering.

It is good to really spend time with this portion of the practice—to truly open up and receive these blessings. This is especially important when you feel a lack of love, or are torn up by despair and fear, or anxious that some things you might have done or said are unforgiveable, or struggle to forgive others.

At the end of the practice, imagine that your entire being is completely healed by the light streaming from this presence. Every single cell of your body has transformed and dissolved into a small sphere of light. This sphere now soars up into the sky and merges inseparably with the heart of the presence you have been visualizing. Take time to rest in this state of oneness for as long as possible before you conclude the meditation.

How do you do Essential Phowa for someone else? The steps are basically the same. The only difference is that you visualize the embodiment of truth, wisdom, and compassion above the head of the person who is suffering or dying. From the depth of your heart, ask for guidance and support for the person. Then imagine rays of light pouring from the presence down to the person. His or her entire being is enveloped by the healing light and gradually transformed by it. By the end, the person dissolves into light and becomes one with the heart of the radiant presence.

Truthfully, I had doubts about how "little me" could possibly offer this kind of spiritual support to anyone. The idea sounded rather grandiose and lofty. When I asked Rinpoche about these doubts, he told me that Khandro Tsering Chodron, his aunt and one of the greatest female practitioners of recent times, had said that one does not have to be a holy man or woman for this practice to be effective. Because of the depth of our connection and our caring for the person, the practice is certain to be of benefit.

One of the very first times I tried the practice of Essential Phowa was with an elderly woman, Mary, who was a devout Christian. As death drew near, she had grown more and more anxious. One evening I was sitting at her bedside. She was visibly upset. "Jesus does not love me. Jesus does not love me," she kept repeating, tears streaming down her pale face. At the most vulnerable time of her life, she felt utterly bereft of her most important source of strength and refuge. "Mary, Jesus loves you. That is his nature. Jesus loves you," I found myself saying gently to her. "Mary, Jesus loves you."

A few nights later, Mary was actively dying. I sat at her side, a bit at a loss as to what to offer her, so I silently began the practice of Essential Phowa. I decided to visualize Jesus in radiant, golden light above her bed. Her breath was labored and there was a feeling of restlessness hanging over the entire room. As I continued to do the practice, she appeared to grow more and more peaceful, and so did the environment. At the actual moment of her death, she took three long breaths. "Mary, Jesus loves you," I said softly and slowly. She seemed already so far away and gone, probably unable to hear my words, yet to my amazement I heard a soft, barely audible "Yes" as she exhaled her final breath.

Utter silence in the room. She was gone. An incredible peace enveloped the space. All I could do was continue to invoke and be with her, in awe of the mystery of what we call death.

I often get asked about the best time to prepare for death. The person asking the question usually already knows the answer—an answer most of us do not want to hear—that preparing for death begins right now, this very moment. We cannot wait for later, because *later* may never happen. We do need to train our busy monkey-like mind and learn to become more and more present, in the pure awareness of the here and now. If we don't train the mind to not be distracted, we could easily miss the opportunity to fully participate in what unfolds at the moment of death. At death, according to certain Buddhist teachings, the ordinary, thinking mind driven by anger, desire, and ignorance dies, and what is laid bare is the true essence of mind, beyond thoughts and emotions. If we recognize this essence, liberation is possible. This essence is likened to the quality and experience of a cloudless sky—open, clear, and spacious. Christian contemplatives and many mystical traditions have different names for this deeper reality of our being. In Buddhism, it is called buddha nature, the nature of our mind, the ground luminosity, or clear light.

Being in Mary's presence at the moment of her death and in the moments following her death, and feeling the profound peace, warmth, and clarity in the room, I wondered if she had caught a glimpse of what practitioners over the ages have experienced.

As professionals who work with the dying, there is always the danger of becoming blasé. We might witness two or three deaths in a week, or even in a day. Imbuing care with spiritual awareness can connect us back to our original intention—to *why* we care. "That connection of being present to another's pain and my role in trying to alleviate it is why I am a doctor," Peter Brown, another graduate of our program, once said. "I have the opportunity to make my occupation a spiritual practice. More than just patching someone up, it's about allowing the true essence that comes from my heart to shine forward."

Over the years I have come to realize that when we invoke a loving and understanding presence we are, in fact, evoking our own qualities that have been always and reliably present within us. The *outer* presence we visualize is only a reflection of our *inner* source for wisdom and compassion. We are actually not separate from the qualities of the presence we call upon in Essential Phowa, or in any contemplative practice for that matter. Visualizing an outer presence of an embodiment of whatever truth we believe in, either in the form of a spiritual figure, radiant light, or simply connecting on a feeling level, can thus be a skillful method to center ourselves and reconnect and relax back into the best aspect of our being. Christina Puchalski, a pioneer in spirituality and medicine, said in a talk given to students at George Washington University, "Being a compassionate presence means connecting to the sacred in another from the sacred place within us."

Dying can be messy. Everything we have not dealt with in life, we are confronted with in death. There is often unfinished business and complex family dynamics we may have pushed away, not to mention spiritual, emotional, and mental distress, physical pain, social isolation, and economic worries. Essential Phowa is not about sugarcoating these realities. Spiritual awareness in caring for another is not about manipulating or sanitizing a situation into something nice, clean, and ultimately "uplifting" and "meaningful." If we practice with this kind of expectation, it won't work. We will be disappointed.

Essential Phowa has encouraged me to let go of my fantasies of what *should* happen and be open to what *needs* to happen, which often turns out to be way beyond what I could have imagined possible. It has taught me to surrender to something vaster than myself and yet feel more connected to my true self. It has taught me to let go and, paradoxically, never to give up.

Some years ago, I was caring for a Chinese woman who only spoke Mandarin. Her seventeen-year-old daughter came to see her every day. During these visits her daughter would stand at the end of her mother's bed and only sit next to her dying mother when we encouraged her to do so. The mother's and daughter's helplessness and grief were palpable, yet they never spoke a word or had any physical contact. Our social worker and the rest of the staff tried hard to find ways to connect them and allow them to say their goodbyes.

At the time I was working night shifts, and when the hospital had quieted down I always tried to sit with the mother and offer the practice of Essential Phowa. I often simply stayed with the invocation, asking help for mother and daughter to find a way back to each other, and for myself to allow their process to happen the way they needed it to. During one of my nightly visits, the mother sang a Chinese song in a low, tender, and sad voice. The melody was simple and beautiful, and I started to hum along while continuing with the practice. Over the next few weeks, every time I visited her she made it her mission to teach me her song. With great patience and stubborn insistence, she taught me the words—every single syllable—correcting me and sometimes scolding me with a playful frown on her face as she listened to my poor pronunciation of Mandarin.

The social worker managed to record her song and gave the tape to the daughter on the morning her mother died. As it turned out, the song was an old Chinese folk song from the village in rural China where the mother had come from so many years ago. The song was about the natural beauty of the place and the longing to go back home. In her own way, through this song, her mother had found a way to connect with her daughter and to say goodbye—even though they never quite had the moving scene we might have imagined for them.

The practice of Essential Phowa has become a quiet backdrop for my work, something that now feels quite ordinary and natural. I do it before I go and visit someone, and whenever I remember it during the day I tune back in to it.

As people approach death, their mental receptivity and sensitivity can dramatically increase. As their hearts and minds are in some sense less contained by their bodies, their minds can become almost atmospheric. Entering a dying person's room can sometimes feel like walking straight into that person's mind. What we bring into the room—our thoughts and feelings—can have a tremendous impact, positively or negatively. If we feel anxious, this feeling becomes part of the other's experience. Likewise, if we feel inspired and open. The more we can cultivate a clear, open, and relaxed mind, the more effective we will be, even perhaps on the most profound level.

I've learned to do the practice quickly, particularly in a crisis situation. In *Facing Death and Finding Hope*, Christine Longaker, a colleague and friend of mine, shares the story of David, an emergency-room doctor in a major city hospital, and the benefits his spiritual practice brings to his work.

> Families panic at the time of death, call 911, and bring their loved one to the emergency room to die. When they arrive, they're not prepared for what is about to happen. What I usually see is enormous fear, confusion, anxiety, and helplessness. The way I used to deal with the situation was through detachment. Outside of doing the best for my patients, I figured there was no way I could impact their situation at all. Telling a family that their loved one has died or is dying was one of the things I hated most about my job. Often the family reacted to me with hostility and anger. Since I started doing this practice in the emergency room, I've watched a person's expression in the final few minutes of life change from fear and anxiety to acceptance, sometimes even a gentle smile. It looks like an opening, a release. Then, when I have to go and tell a family that their loved one has died, I notice an enormous difference in their reaction. Family members often thank me and even come up and hug me. This new experience I am having since doing my spiritual practice in the hospital has transformed my life and my medical practice.

We may never come to see the effects of our care in such tangible ways, yet every gesture of kindness and courage is of benefit. Every time we extend ourselves to another we have the chance to connect to a deeper dimension of life. Care founded on spiritual awareness always embraces the fullness of the human experience. We are all imperfect and vulnerable, *and* we are all fundamentally good and whole. The latter we often lose sight of or tend to neglect.

Of course, Essential Phowa is a poignant reminder to be ready for the moment of death ourselves. To be with the dying is to be with our *own* dying. It is an incredible opportunity if, instead of continuously turning away from the fear, we can learn through practices such as Essential Phowa to mindfully turn toward it. The transformative power and adaptability of this practice still amazes me, and I feel I have a long way to go to fully grasp its depth and meaning.

Essential Phowa, based on my own experience and listening to others' stories, has the power to connect us back to *the heart of care* and to the best aspect of ourselves—the one that is fundamentally sane, healthy, courageous, and good. Essential Phowa can help transform being with the dying into a deeply meaningful, even sacred task. It transforms the process of dying into a sacred journey, and death from just a medical event into a sacred moment.

Our Real Home 17

Ajahn Chah

The following is from a talk addressed to an aging lay disciple approaching her death, as well as to her family and caregivers.

Resolve now to listen respectfully to the Dhamma. While I am speaking, be as attentive to my words as if it were the Lord Buddha himself sitting before you. Close your eyes and make yourself comfortable, composing your mind and making it one-pointed. Humbly allow the Triple Gem of wisdom, truth, and purity to abide in your heart as a way of showing respect to the Fully Enlightened One.

Today I have brought nothing of material substance to offer you, only the Dhamma, the teachings of the Lord Buddha. You should understand that even the Buddha himself, with his great store of accumulated virtue, could not avoid physical death. When he reached old age he ceded his body and let go of the heavy burden. Now you too must learn to be satisfied with the many years you've depended on your body. You should feel that it's enough.

Think of household utensils that you've had for a long time—cups, saucers, plates. When you first got them, they were clean and shining, but now after using them for so long, they're starting to wear out. Some are already broken, some have disappeared, and those that are left are wearing out; they have no enduring form. And it's their nature to be that way. Your body is the same, continually changing from the day you were born, through childhood and youth, until it reaches old age. You must accept this. The Buddha said that conditions, whether internal bodily conditions or external conditions, are not-self; their nature is to change. Contemplate this truth clearly.

This very lump of flesh lying here in decline is reality, *sacca-dhamma.* The facts of this body are reality; they are the timeless teaching of the Lord Buddha. The Buddha taught us to contemplate this and come to terms with its nature. We must be able to be at peace with the body, no matter what state it is in. The Buddha told us that we should ensure that it's only the body that is locked up in jail, and not to let the mind be imprisoned along with it. Now as your body begins to run down and wear out with age, don't resist, but also don't let your mind deteriorate along with it. Keep the mind separate. Give energy to the mind by realizing the truth of the way things are. The Lord Buddha taught that this is the nature of the body; it can't be any other way. Having been born it gets old and sick and then it dies. This is a great truth that you are presently witnessing. Look at the body with wisdom and realize this.

If your house is flooded or burned to the ground, allow that threat to affect only the house. If there's a flood, don't let it flood your mind. If there's a fire, don't let it burn your heart. Let it be merely the house—which is outside—that is flooded or burned. Now is the time to allow the mind to let go of attachments.

You've been alive a long time now. Your eyes have seen any number of forms and colors, your ears have heard so many sounds, you've had any number of experiences. And that's all they were—experiences. You've eaten delicious foods, and all those good tastes were just good tastes, nothing more. The bad tastes were just bad tastes, that's all. If the eye sees a beautiful form, that's all it is—a beautiful form. An ugly form is just an ugly form. The ear hears an entrancing, melodious sound, and it's nothing more than that. A grating, discordant sound is simply that.

The Buddha said that rich or poor, young or old, human or animal, no being in this world can maintain itself in any single state for long. Everything experiences change and deprivation. This is a fact of life we cannot remedy. But the Buddha said that what we can do is contemplate the body and mind to see their impersonality, to see that neither of them is "me" nor "mine." They have only a provisional reality. Like your house, it's only nominally yours. You couldn't take it with you anywhere. The same applies to your wealth, your possessions, and your family—they're yours only in name. They don't really belong to you; they belong to nature.

Now this truth doesn't apply to you alone; everyone is in the same boat—even the Lord Buddha and his enlightened disciples. They differed from us only in one respect, and that was their acceptance of the way things are. They saw that it could be no other way.

So the Buddha asked us to probe and examine the body, from the soles of the feet up to the crown of the head, and then back down to the feet again. Just take a look at the body. What sort of things do you see? Is there anything intrinsically clean there? Can you find any abiding essence? This whole body is steadily degenerating. The Buddha taught us to see that it doesn't belong to us. It's natural for the body to be this way, because all conditioned phenomena are subject to change. How else would you have it? In fact there is nothing wrong with the way the body is. It's not the body that causes suffering; it's wrong thinking. When you see things the wrong way, there's bound to be confusion.

It's like a river. Water naturally flows downhill. That's nature. If a person were to go and stand on the river bank and want the water to flow back uphill, they would be foolish. Wherever they went, their foolish thinking would allow them no peace of mind. They would suffer because of their wrong view, for their thinking goes against the stream. If they had right view, they would see that the water must inevitably flow downhill, and until they realized and accepted that fact, they would be bewildered and frustrated.

The river that must flow down a slope is like your body. Once young, your body's become old and is meandering toward death. Don't go wishing it were otherwise; it's not something you have the power to remedy. The Buddha told us to see the way things are and then let go of our clinging to them. Take this feeling of letting go as your refuge.

Look upon the in- and out-breaths as if they were relatives who come to visit you. When the relatives leave, you follow them out to see them off. You watch until they've walked up the drive and out of sight, and then you go back indoors. We watch the breath in the same way. If the breath is coarse, we know that it's coarse; if it's subtle, we know that.

So let go, put everything down, everything except the knowing. Don't be fooled if visions or sounds arise in your mind during meditation. Lay them all down. Don't take hold of anything at all. Just stay with this unified awareness. Don't worry about the past or the future; just be still and you will reach the place where there's no advancing, no retreating, and no stopping, where there's nothing to grasp at or cling to. Why? Because there's no self, no "me" or "mine." It's all gone. The Buddha taught us to be emptied of everything in this way, not to carry anything around. To know, and having known, let go.

Realizing the Dhamma, the path to freedom from the round of birth and death, is a task that we all have to do alone. So keep trying to let go and understand the teachings. Put effort into your contemplation. Don't worry about your family. At the moment they are as they are; in the future they will be like you. There's no one in the world who can escape this fate. The Buddha taught us to lay down those things that lack a real abiding essence. If you lay everything down you will see the truth; if you don't, you won't. That's the way it is. And it's the same for everyone in the world. So don't grasp at anything.

If you find yourself thinking, well, that's all right too, as long as you think wisely. Whatever the mind turns to, think about it with wisdom, be aware of its nature. If you know something with wisdom, you let it go and there's no suffering. The mind is bright, joyful, and at peace. It turns away from distractions and is undivided. Right now what you can look to for help and support is your breath.

Thinking you'd like to go on living for a long time will make you suffer. But thinking you'd like to die soon or right away isn't right either. It's suffering, isn't it? Conditions don't belong to us, they follow their own natural laws. You can't do anything about the way the body is. But what you can improve and beautify is the mind.

Anyone can build a house of wood and bricks, but that sort of home, the Buddha taught, is not our real home, it's only nominally ours. It's a home in the world and it follows the ways of the world. Our real home is inner peace. An external, material home may well be pretty, but it is not very peaceful—there's this worry and then that—so we may say it's not our real home, it's external to us. Sooner or later we'll have to give it up. It's not a place we can live in permanently because it doesn't truly belong to us; it belongs to the world. Our body is the same. We take it to be a self, to be "me" or "mine," but in fact it's not really so at all; it's another worldly home. Your body has followed its natural course from birth, and now it's old and sick. You can't forbid it from doing that. That's the way it is. Wanting it to be different would be as foolish as wanting a duck to be like a chicken. When you see that that's impossible—that a duck must be a duck and a chicken must be a chicken, and the bodies have to get old and die—you will find courage and energy. However much you want the body to go on lasting, it won't do that.

The Buddha said,

Aniccā vata saṅkhārā
Uppāda vaya dhammino
Uppajjitvā nirujjhan 'ti
Tesam vūpasamo sukho

Impermanent are all conditioned things
Of the nature to arise and pass away
Having been born, they all must cease
The calming of conditions is true happiness

The word *saṅkhāra* refers to this body and mind. *Saṅkhārās* are impermanent and unstable. Having come into being they disappear, having arisen they pass away, and yet everyone wants them to be permanent. This is foolishness. Look at the breath. Having come in, it goes out; that's its nature, that's how it has to be. The inhalations and exhalations have to alternate, there must be change. Conditions exist through change; you can't prevent it. Just think, could you exhale without inhaling? Would it feel good? Or could you just inhale? We want things to be permanent but they can't be; it's impossible. Once the breath has come in, it must go out. When it's out, it comes back in again, and that's natural, isn't it? Having been born we get old and then die, and that's totally natural and normal. It's because conditions have done their job, because the in-breaths and out-breaths have alternated in this way, that the human race is still here today.

As soon as we are born, we are dead. Our birth and our death are just one thing. It's like a tree: when there's a root there must be branches. When there are branches there must be a root. You can't have one without the other. It's a little funny to see how at death people are so grief-stricken and distracted, and at birth how happy and delighted. It's delusion; nobody has ever looked at this clearly. I think if you really want to cry, it would be better to do so when someone's born. Birth is death, death is birth; the branch is the root, the root is the branch. If you must cry, cry at the root; cry at the birth. Look closely: If there were no birth, there would be no death. Can you understand this?

Don't worry about things too much; just think, "This is the way things are." This is your work, your duty. Right now nobody can help you, there's nothing that your family and possessions can do for you. All that can help you now is clear awareness.

So don't waver. Let go. Throw it all away.

Even if you don't let go, everything is starting to leave you anyway. Can you see that, how all the different parts of your body are trying to slip away? Take your hair; when you were young it was thick and black. Now it's falling out. It's leaving. Your eyes used to be good and strong but now they're weak; your sight is unclear. When your organs have had enough they leave, for this isn't their home. When you were a child your teeth were healthy and firm; now they're wobbly, or you've got false ones. Your eyes, ears, nose, tongue—everything is trying to leave because this isn't their home. You can't make a permanent home in conditions; you can only stay for a short time and then you have to go. It's like a tenant watching over his tiny house with failing eyes. His teeth aren't so good, his eyes aren't so good, his body's not so healthy; everything is leaving.

So you needn't worry about anything, because this isn't your real home; it's only a temporary shelter. Having come into this world, you should contemplate its nature. Everything is preparing to disappear. Look at your body. Is there anything there that's still in its original form? Is your skin as it used to be? Is your hair? They aren't the same, are they? Where has everything gone? This is nature, the way things are. When their time is up, conditions go their way. In this world there is nothing to rely on—it's an endless round of disturbance and trouble, pleasure and pain. There is no peace.

When we have no real home we're like aimless travelers out on the road, going here and there, stopping for a while and then setting off again. Until we return to our real homes we feel uneasy, just like a villager who's left their village. Only when they get home can they really relax and be at peace.

Nowhere in the world is there any real peace to be found. The poor have no peace and neither do the rich; adults have no peace and neither do children; the poorly educated have no peace and neither do the highly educated. There's no peace anywhere; that's the nature of the world. Those who have few possessions suffer, and so do those who have many. Children, adults, the aged, everyone suffers. The suffering of being old, the suffering of being young, the suffering of being wealthy, and the suffering of being poor—it's all nothing but suffering.

When you've contemplated things in this way you'll see *anicca*, impermanence, and *dukkha*, unsatisfactoriness. Why are things impermanent and unsatisfactory? Because they are *anattā*, not-self.

Both your body that is lying sick and in pain, and the mind that is aware of its sickness and pain, are called *dhamma*. That which is formless—the thoughts, feelings, and perceptions—is called *nāmadhamma.* That which is racked with aches and pain is called *rūpadhamma.* The material is dhamma and the immaterial is dhamma. So we live *with* dhammas, *in* dhammas, and we *are* dhammas. In truth, there is no self to be found; there are only dhammas continually arising and passing away. Every single moment we're undergoing birth and death. This is the way things are.

When we think of the Lord Buddha, how truly he spoke, we feel how worthy he is of reverence and respect. Whenever we see the truth of something, we see his teachings, even if we've never actually practiced the Dhamma. But even if we have a knowledge of the teachings and have studied and practiced them, as long as we still haven't seen the truth we are still homeless.

So understand this point. All people, all creatures, are preparing to leave. When beings have lived an appropriate time, they must go on their way. Rich, poor, young, and old must all experience this change.

When you realize that's the way the world is, you'll feel that it's a wearisome place. When you see that there's nothing real or substantial you can rely on, you'll feel weary and disenchanted. Being disenchanted doesn't mean you are averse; the mind is clear. It sees that there's nothing to be done to remedy this state of affairs; it's just the way the world is. Knowing in this way you can let go of attachment, letting go with a mind that is neither happy nor sad, but at peace with conditions through seeing their changing nature with wisdom. *Aniccā vata saṅkhārā*—all conditions are impermanent.

Impermanence is the Buddha. If we truly see an impermanent condition, we see that it's permanent—in the sense that its subjection to change is unchanging. This is the permanence that living beings possess: continual transformation from childhood through to old age, and that very impermanence, that propensity to change, is permanent and fixed. If you look at it like this your heart will be at ease. When you consider things in this way you'll see them as wearisome, and disenchantment will arise. Your delight in the world of sense pleasures will disappear. You'll see that if you have many possessions, you have to leave a lot behind. If you have few, you leave few behind. Wealth is just wealth, long life is just long life. They're nothing special.

What is important is that we should do as the Lord Buddha taught and build our own home, building it by the method that I've been explaining to you. Build your own home. Let go. Let go until the mind reaches the peace that is free from advancing, free from retreating, and free from stopping still. Pleasure is not your home, pain is not your home. Pleasure and pain both decline and pass away.

The Buddha saw that all conditions are impermanent, so he taught us to let go of our attachment to them. When we reach the end of our life we'll have no choice anyway. So wouldn't it be better to put things down before then? They're just a heavy burden to carry around; why not throw off that load now?

Let go.

Relax.

For the Anniversary of My Death

W. S. Merwin

Every year without knowing it I have passed the day
When the last fires will wave to me
And the silence will set out
Tireless traveler
Like the beam of a lightless star

Then I will no longer
Find myself in life as in a strange garment
Surprised at the earth
And the love of one woman
And the shamelessness of men
As today writing after three days of rain
Hearing the wren sing and the falling cease
And bowing not knowing to what

Separation

W. S. Merwin

Your absence has gone through me
Like thread through a needle.
Everything I do is stitched with its color.

Don't Wait for Tomorrow: Six Meditations on Death and Dying 18

Stephen and Ondrea Levine

No One Should Die Alone

If possible, no one should die alone. A hand held can sometimes bring more relief than a strong analgesic. Always remember that the person in the sick bed should be listened to very closely so as to know what they want most. They are the captain of the boat they have been building their whole life to cross the great waters.

Forgiveness

Forgiveness can finish unfinished business. But it takes a while to cultivate the openness of heart necessary to allow a lifetime's armoring to gradually disintegrate—to allow the fist around the heart to loosen and let go of unattended sorrows. Sometimes in the course of listening to a loved one's life review, elements of unfinished business may surface and make themselves vulnerable to healing.

Sometimes it can help to write a letter about one's unfinished business as a way of untangling the loose ends over which we so often trip. We have seen people then burn that letter as a way to let go, forgive, or say goodbye.

Don't wait for death to remind you to live. Death is a perfect mirror for life. It clarifies priorities. It will point out the way to the heart: compassion and loving-kindness, generosity and courage.

In response to the Dalai Lama asking me what I was working on,

I told him I was writing a book called *A Year to Live* about preparing for death by thoroughly living. He asked, "Would that be skillful with the American consciousness?" I told him that of the thousands of terminally ill people we worked with, received phone calls from, and exchanged letters with, none had ever chosen to grab a bottle of tequila and a sex partner and head for the hills. He laughed and shook his head. "Very good, very good," he said. "Preparing for death has for millennia been recommended as a precise teaching and practice for cultivating wisdom and mercy."

Regret

Many of those we have accompanied during their last days and hours died in relative peace. Some died with considerable regret.

The most common theme of regret was a feeling that the person had given their life away to a job they did not care about instead of toward some work they loved. People wished they had gotten a job for the love of it and not for the money. One lawyer said he wished he had gotten into furniture design—he loved the smooth even beat of his heart at the whirring lathe. Another—a very successful Broadway set designer, who was also autistic—wished he had become an accountant because the numbers helped straighten his mind.

The second most common area of regret had to do with relationships. Some wished they had gotten a divorce instead of staying with their partner out of fear and uncertainty. Others wished they had gotten married. Some wished they had been different or better parents. More than a few wished they had put more work into opening their heart and been less stubborn, less self-protective. Many wished they had spent more time playing, making love, or serving the needs of others.

Don't Wait for Tomorrow to Live

Pretense is the first thing to fall away as the energy gathers in the heart and the body beings to loose itself of fear. Don't wait for tomorrow. No one has ever lived a tomorrow. Only being present in the present leads to a life well lived.

Love as Ombudsman

We have repeatedly observed that those who forgive the most profoundly seem to heal the deepest. Love is a gatekeeper that, unlike most, struggles to keep the gate open.

What We Took Birth For

We have witnessed moments of almost blinding spirit. We have been engulfed in a peace that went well beyond understanding. We have experienced the hard work of caregivers under dire circumstances and the grace that often met their efforts, as well as the effortless unfolding of what might be called miracles. The deathbed can sometimes make manifest the extraordinary depths of the human heart.

We have seen some who had lived mean-spirited, unkind, even violent lives have unexpectedly beautiful, peaceful, and merciful deaths. And we have seen people die very much as they have lived.

There are parts of us that know us better than we do. Just below the level of awareness is the primal knowing that what passes into death and comes out the other end is our essential nature. In our original nature lies the beginning of the world. The love and fear that drives us to take birth, that draws the next breath, opens to the healing we took birth for.

Sunao

Spitting blood
clears up reality
and dream alike.

19
A Lesson in Compassion

Betsy MacGregor

When I completed four grueling years of medical school, stuffing my head full of scientific knowledge, and finally donned the white coat that identified me as a real doctor, I had no idea I was entering my pediatric internship in the middle of an epidemic, or that that epidemic would teach me more about compassion than all my spiritual studies combined. It was 1976, and AIDS was slamming my beloved New York City with devastating force. Little was yet known about this new virus that attacked the human immune system so viciously, only that pitifully little could be done to help those unfortunate enough to be infected with it. And sadly, the ones who were proving to be most vulnerable to the virus tended to be those who lived in the inner-city neighborhoods where life was hard enough already, burdened as it was with poor housing conditions, inadequate education, drug abuse, violence, broken family bonds, and lack of opportunity. These were the neighborhoods my hospital served and where the children I would care for were growing up.

We admitted a great number of children who were sick with AIDS to my hospital back in those days, and sadly we lost many of them. One two-year-old boy I remember in particular. As was typical, he had acquired the virus from his infected mother when he was born, and despite our best efforts to help him, he was slowly slipping away from us. He lay quietly in his crib, hollow-eyed and emaciated, never smiling or even crying. He simply did not have the energy.

The little boy's mother had brought him to our emergency room one night, burning up with fever. The chest x-ray we took showed he had pneumonia, and so we promptly admitted him to the pediatric ward. His mother lingered at his side for a time, but then departed and never returned. Eventually we learned she had been admitted to another hospital shortly after leaving ours and had died there from complications of her own AIDS. The one thing she had left her son was his name. She had called him Angel.

Angel had been on our pediatric ward for three months. There was no other place that wanted him, and frankly we were happy to keep him with us. At least we knew he would be fed and kept clean and sheltered—and would occasionally be held in another human being's arms, when one of the staff was able to spare a moment or two. We knew he had little time left.

One night, when I was on call and kept busy on the ward into the wee hours of the night, I glimpsed a side of Angel's story I had not been aware of before. The ward's lights had all been turned down and most of the children put to sleep in their beds, and I was going about the typical work of an intern—reviewing orders, checking on patients' vital signs, and peeking in on the sickest ones—when something caught my ear. A faint lyrical sound was whispering down one of the dimly lit hallways. Listening closely, I detected the thin notes of a melody carried by a human voice.

I was tired and still had chores to do, but the wistful sound called to me, and so I followed it. It led me to Angel's room. Yet what I saw through the doorway as I approached made me pause and remain in the quiet shadows of the hallway rather than enter. For it was clear that more was taking place in Angel's room than the sad wasting of an unfulfilled life. Something more intimate was happening, something that needed not to be disturbed.

With Angel was his father. I had never seen the man before, but I'd heard from the other staff that he often came in the wee hours of the night to visit his son. He was a tough-looking person, unshaven and stamped with the harsh signs of inner city life and his own battle with AIDS.

The man was sitting in a chair, holding Angel on his lap and feeding him infant formula with a dropper. As I watched, he waited carefully for his son's lips to accept each drop before offering him another, all the while gazing into his child's eyes and softly crooning a melody—a hauntingly soothing sound, the notes filled with reassurance and encouragement. Angel's eyes remained fastened on his father's face, as if he were drinking in life-giving nourishment from the look that he saw there.

The two of them were in such a rapt communion that I remained bound in unmoving silence outside their door. It seemed that I had been summoned not to enter, but to stand as an observer of this exquisite scene.

What I had been called to witness, my heart said, was the compassion that was shining brightly in that little room. Nothing more than that, and nothing less. In the light of that compassion, the tragedy of Angel's pitiful life—of both their lives—was being lifted up and set aside. I could feel the truth of that as surely as anything my medical books had ever taught me.

The shadows in the hallway seemed to whisper: *Do you see? This is what compassion is. It is a force more powerful than even life-destroying disease. It can willingly embrace whatever the world has abandoned as hopeless and transform it into something to be cherished.*

As I dropped my eyes and turned to go back to work, gratitude for having glimpsed this side of Angel's story filled me. I could not help but wonder: how many of us will be sung to with that much compassion as we lie in our own last days of life?

A Bowl

Rumi, translated by Coleman Barks

Imagine the time the particle you are
returns where it came from!

The family darling comes home. Wine,
without being contained in cups,
is handed around.

A red glint appears in a granite outcrop,
and suddenly the whole cliff turns to ruby.

At dawn I walked along with a monk
on his way to the monastery.
                                        "We do the same work,"
I told him. "We suffer the same."

He gave me a bowl.
And I saw:
        The soul has *this* shape.
                                        Shams,
you that teach us and actual sunlight,
                                        help me now,

Being in the middle of being partly in my self,
and partly outside.

Bird Wings

Rumi, translated by Coleman Barks

Your grief for what you've lost lifts a mirror up to
where you're bravely working.

Expecting the worst, you look, and instead,
Here's the joyful face you've been wanting to see.

Your hand opens and closes and opens and closes.
If it were always a fist or always stretched open,
you would be paralyzed.

Your deepest presence is in every small contracting
and expanding,
the two as beautifully balanced and coordinated
as birdwings.

The Guest House

Rumi, translated by Coleman Barks

This being human is a guest house.
Every morning a new arrival.

A joy, a depression, a meanness,
some momentary awareness comes
as an unexpected visitor.

Welcome and entertain them all!
Even if they are a crowd of sorrows,
who violently sweep your house
empty of its furniture,
still, treat each guest honorably.
He may be clearing you out
for some new delight.

The dark thought, the shame, the malice,
meet them at the door laughing,
and invite them in.

Be grateful for whoever comes,
because each has been sent
as a guide from beyond.

The Third Messenger: Death Is Unavoidable

20

Larry Rosenberg

In brief, without being mindful of death, whatever Dharma practices you take up will be merely superficial.
—Milarepa

We know in our heads that we will die. But we have to know it in our hearts. We have to let this fact penetrate our bones. Then we will know how to live.

To do that, we need to be able to look at the fact of death with steadiness. We can't just glance at it casually. All of our training in Dharma practice is preparation for such deep seeing. Taking the refuges and ethical precepts, which is a traditional first step; working with the breath—which can be a long process—to develop a calm and concentrated mind; working with sensations, with small fears and progressively larger ones; developing mindfulness in everyday life: All of these steps work together to build a mind that is strong enough to look at the fear of death. Sometimes, before we are able to observe this fear directly, we need to learn how to be with our resistance to it. We are mindful of how much we hate to have fear in the first place.

If you haven't done this preparatory work, you probably aren't going to be ready to look at death. There may be a few exceptional individuals who can, who just seem to arrive on the earth with remarkable spiritual maturity or who have perhaps had life experiences that develop that maturity. But most of us need to work at it. We need to develop a mind that is capable of looking at things with some steadiness, so we can stay with them long enough for the message to come through. Communing with fear stimulates an understanding that has liberating power.

Typically, our awareness is sporadic. We might be watching the evening news and hear some tragedy, and we notice a momentary pang or a real feeling of heartsickness. But something else comes on the screen, or we move on to some other activity, and it's over. That's the way of the modern world. Short brief bursts of attention.

Our practice is different. The *samadhi* we develop is not a rigid attention, which shuts things out. The mind that develops samadhi is strong and supple, very much alive. The state we develop is more like tenderness. The heart begins to melt. You see the true sorrow of life and its true beauty. You can't see one without the other. Practice opens us up to both.

Sometimes when your heart grows tender from practice, a single event touches it in such a way that you are suddenly more awake: You see deeply into the nature of things. Then everything becomes more precious, all of the people and all of the surroundings of your life. Your urge to intensify meditation practice can grow as well.

I don't mean something narrow by practice, that you quit your job and leave your family to go off and meditate in a cave somewhere. I mean it in a broad sense: You stay awake in everything you do. You make the practice a vital part of your entire life. And when you learn to practice with ordinary events, you are capable of staying with the extraordinary ones. Like the moment of death.

I have learned a great deal from the teachings of Zen Master Suzuki Shosan, a meditator who had also been a samurai and who had even put in some time as a hermit. He had been fiercely trained in combat. His teaching was to use death awareness or, as he put it, "death energy," to stimulate his practice. When problems came up in his life, he would use death energy to reorchestrate the conditions, and it proved to be a great help.

"If you yourself can die gladly," he said, "you will have become a Buddha. Buddhahood is to die with an easy mind." He goes on, with painful honesty: "Because I am a man who does not want to die, I practice in order to be able to die freely. Freely stretching out my neck for the executioner without a thought."

He is using the executioner as a symbol of death. He means that when the time comes, he hopes to surrender to death gracefully. "I've trained myself in various ways," he says, "and I know the agony of not dying freely. My method is a coward's Buddhism." We are all cowards, in that sense. We all need some kind of training.

Some of the deepest learning about death is not formal, of course; it comes about naturally when—for instance—one's parents die. But you learn from such an event only if you really look at it, as you would in more formal practice. If you're open to the experience, every person who dies is your teacher.

I feel that my father's last gift to me was that he taught me I was going to die. I'm not exempt from the law he was subject to. I have had moments in my life when it seemed unthinkable that my father would die, this man who for many years seemed bigger and stronger than I and who I modeled myself on when I was growing up. But he did die, and he's not coming back. Ashes do not become wood again. Someday I too will be ashes.

Practicing Formally

These thoughts about my father actually begin to move us into more formal death awareness practices. I have used—and taught—a nine-part meditation that has been adapted from the teaching of Atisha (980–1055), the great Indian Buddhist sage. I have modified these contemplations with personal instructions from Tara Tulku Rinpoche and Ajaan Suwat. They are the basis of the death meditations that I teach today.

This practice is divided into three general topics: the inevitability of death, the uncertainty of when we will die, and the fact that nothing but the Dharma can help you at the time of death. Each category includes three contemplations.

In a typical session, it is a good idea to begin with breath awareness, giving the breath exclusive attention until the mind settles down. Once you have reached some calm, you are ready to take up a contemplation like the first one: Everyone must die.

Obviously, this contemplation requires a concentrated mind. There is no fact of human existence that we are more likely to want to escape. We naturally have great aversion to it, and when our capacity to pay attention is limited the true significance of the contemplation does not penetrate to the heart. But in a serene mind, thinking can be sharp and pliable. We can direct our attention with precision and focus, and our reflection can be uninterrupted. It has the powerful support of samadhi, which enables us to stay emotionally engaged and keenly interested.

If we just turn the contemplation over in our mind, the richness of its meaning reveals itself. We stay attentive to our experience as it tells its story and allow the truth of the contemplation to affect us. We experience it not just with our thinking mind but with our entire being. These nine reflections of Atisha are an exercise in *yoniso manasikara*—careful concentration. Any of these simple verbal statements when attended to in a thorough and sustained way can take us beyond their surface meaning. Probing these statements deeply can help us uncover the workings of the natural law of Dharma in our own bodies and minds.

In a given session, you might give your primary focus to a particular contemplation, then briefly review the other eight to remind yourself of them. You might choose to do one contemplation per day, or perhaps all three within a particular heading. If a given contemplation seems fruitful, you might want to stay with it for a number of days. All of these contemplations get at the same basic truth, and your practice with them need not be rigid. You can use your innate wisdom to decide how best to work with them.

All of this will become clearer as we move into specific examples.

The Inevitability of Death

I. Everyone must die.

The first—and boldest—of these contemplations is that everyone and everything must die. No one escapes this inevitable law. Death is a logical consequence of birth and begins to work on life at the moment of birth. There are no exceptions. Differences in wealth, education, physical strength, fame, moral integrity, even spiritual maturity, are irrelevant. If you don't want to die, don't be born.

Buddhaghosha's *Visuddhimagga* is of some help here. It suggests that you compare yourself with others of great fame, merit, supernatural powers, deep understanding. The Buddha died. Jesus Christ. Socrates. Great and famous athletes: the strongest men and women in the world, the fastest, those capable of the most extraordinary physical feats.

I often contemplate Krishnamurti in this way. It is helpful if you have actually known the person. He had incredible inner strength and clarity and immense vitality, which I experienced in his presence over a period of many years. He taught until several weeks before he died at the age of ninety. But he did die.

You can also take up ordinary people who have seemed extremely vital and alive. Probably we have all known someone who seemed absolutely irrepressible and unstoppable. That person, too, is subject to death.

Sometimes methods just suggest themselves. One night some years ago I had given a talk on death awareness, so it was on my mind afterward when I went up to my apartment to unwind. I love movies, especially old ones. That night there was a film from 1938 with Clark Gable and Carole Lombard, and as a film buff I had heard of everyone involved, the writer, the director, the producer. Suddenly I realized that everyone connected with that movie was dead.

There they were bounding around in the prime of life, wonderfully virile and sensual and attractive. And all of them were dead. The person who got the idea, the person who fleshed it out and wrote the screenplay, the person who wrote the score—everyone who played in the orchestra. Probably even the people who sold the popcorn in the theatres were dead. It was stunning to realize. The movie was so alive, and they were so dead.

The Buddha put it this way [in the Mahaparinibbana Sutta]:

> Young and old,
> foolish and wise,
> rich and poor,
> all keep dying.
> As a potter's clay vessels,
> large and small,
> fired and unfired,
> all end up broken,
> so too life leads to death.

2. The remainder of our lifespan is decreasing continually.

Our movement toward death is inexorable. It never stops. From the moment we're born, we are dying. Death comes closer with every tick of the clock. The great Indian master Atisha used the sound of dripping water as a way to practice this contemplation.

We can use a variety of objects. One of the simplest—and best—is the breath itself. We have only a finite number of breaths in our life—it may be a rather large number, of course, and we have no idea what it is—and with each breath we use up another. Every breath brings us closer to death.

This is part of the real depth of breath awareness, the place where it can take us. We start out thinking we're watching a simple physical function, but the more we do it, the more we realize what a profound phenomenon we're observing. Each inhalation, after all, is a tiny bit of life; it is bringing air into the lungs, oxygen into the body, and allowing us to live. Each exhalation is a letting go, a releasing. At some point we will exhale and not inhale again. And our life will end.

We can contemplate the breath in exactly that way, releasing each exhalation with no certainty or even expectation that there will be another breath. Especially when we have been sitting for a while, the breath can grow very deep, and there can be a long pause between exhalation and inhalation. It can be a moment that is fraught with anxiety. Sometimes we finally force an inhalation, just to assure ourselves that we will breathe again. But the more we sit, the more we are able to let the process just happen and stay with the moment between breaths, when we are not sure we will breathe again.

Such a practice can sound terrifying. We might be arousing one of our primal fears—the fear that we will not be able to get our breath—which is behind many of our other, smaller fears. And whatever the contemplation calls up—fear, terror, hysteria—that is what we practice with. We stay with it, letting that fear exist alongside the process of the breath itself, and see that it too is an impermanent phenomenon, that it is workable.

Such a fear is very much like physical pain. If we turn away from it or run from it, it looms larger and larger and can become very difficult. But if we stay with it, we see first of all that it isn't as bad as we might have thought. Then we see that it comes to an end. Our whole relationship to fear—and to breathing—can change in that moment. Seeing impermanence helps us decondition the mind's strong tendency to grasp and cling.

Sometimes, of course, we sit down expecting fear to come up, expecting some violent reaction, and nothing happens. Or maybe fear arises briefly and doesn't continue. We keep turning the contemplation over in our minds with no result. That's all right. We can't control such things and can never be sure when our emotions will engage. We don't want to force anything or have the feeling that we're trying to break through to something. We just want to be present with the experience we are having.

In any case, the second contemplation concerns our steadily decreasing number of days. It is as if we have fallen from a tree in the dark of night. We know we're going to hit the ground at some point. We just don't know when. The seventh Dalai Lama expressed it in a poem ["Meditations on the Ways of Impermanence," translated by Glenn Mullin].

> After our birth we have no freedom to remain
> even for a minute.
> We head towards the embrace of the Lord of Death,
> like an athlete running.
> We may think that we are among the living, but our life
> is the very highway of death.

3. Death will come regardless of whether or not we have made time to practice the Dharma.

This contemplation focuses on the fact that our major reason for contemplating death is to spur us on to practice. I assume in that statement a basic commitment to meditation practice, and I may be assuming too much. I am, after all, a meditation teacher. It may be that another kind of person confronting the harsh reality of death might give up his job and opt for a life of sex, drugs, and rock and roll. Who knows?

But this contemplation is letting us know that time is precious and we have little of it. We all spend countless hours sleeping, eating, just hanging around. Not that those things aren't important. But we have to ask ourselves how we want to spend what precious little time we have.

We have all probably asked ourselves: What would I do if I had just one more year to live? It is an interesting question, and we all hope we have more than that, but we definitely have a limited time. How do we want to spend it? To what do we want to devote our lives? It's a question we need to ask.

As a Dharma teacher, I frequently meet people who are wrestling with this contemplation. "As soon as I get my degree, I'm really going to practice." "When I finish my novel . . ." "When I close one last business deal . . ." "When my children are grown . . ." Gungtang Rinpoche summed up this mindset well:

> I spent twenty years not wanting to practice dharma. I spent the next twenty years thinking that I could practice later on. I spent another twenty years in other activities and regretting the fact that I hadn't engaged in the dharma practice. This is the story of my empty human life.

What is really needed here is a change in priorities, as well as a change in attitude. Almost all of us have circumstances in our lives that make practice somewhat difficult. And when people make these excuses to me, they are mostly talking about finding more time for daily sitting practice, more time to do all-day sittings and longer retreats. These things are extremely valuable and important. But the real question is: Do we dare to practice, to commit ourselves to practice, right now? The whole of our lives is a wonderful field of practice. Can we use it? The simplified, protected situation of formal sitting practice is invaluable, but can we also practice while we are raising our children, going to school, going to work, writing a novel, even driving a car or going to the bathroom? The mindset that sees certain periods of time as available for practice and others as not is mistaken from the outset. All of us can practice, with everything we do. It is just a question of whether or not we dare to do it.

When people approach practice in that way, when they bring it into their daily lives, what often happens is that they see benefits from it, and their practice catches fire, and suddenly time for sitting practice looks different. When they come to understand that sitting is the real basis of practice, it is amazing how time suddenly shows up for it. It almost happens by itself.

So the first thing people need to face is not a scheduling conflict. It is whether or not they want to give themselves to practice. When students do that, the time shows up by itself.

This contemplation faces that question directly: To what will we give the days of our lives?

The Uncertainty of the Time of Death

4. Human life expectancy is uncertain.

A graveyard is a wonderful place to practice contemplation, especially an old one. Just walk around and look at the headstones and see at what age people died. But sometimes an old graveyard gives us a false sense of security; we think that since the discovery of antibiotics and of various vaccines, because of all of our recent medical advances, things have changed. They have; the average life expectancy is longer. But people still die at all ages. Just read your newspaper. Watch CNN. Talk to your neighbors. You'll hear all kinds of stories.

This contemplation really just reflects the law of impermanence. A corollary of that law is that change happens in unexpected ways. It would be one thing if all phenomena changed predictably. It might still be difficult, but at least it would have a pattern. But the truth is that life can snatch the rug out from under us. The floor can cave in. So can the roof. And we never know when such an event might happen.

It isn't just death that is uncertain but also life. We all want permanent things: a permanent partner, a permanent job, a permanent family, house, income, group of friends, place to practice meditation. Permanently good weather. We do everything we can to assure permanence in all of these areas; we spend all of our time trying to assure ourselves, and it never works. Nothing is permanent. We would spend our time much more wisely by contemplating and absorbing the law of impermanence rather than trying to repeal it. If we could learn to live with it, our lives would be much different.

It is like the story of a famous sage who was asked where all his wisdom came from. He replied, "I live as a man who, when he wakes up in the morning, does not know if he will be alive when the day ends." His questioners were puzzled. "Isn't that true of everybody?" they asked. "It is," he said, "but few people live that way."

The law of impermanence is not good news or bad news. It isn't even news. It is just a fact, the most obvious fact in the universe. But we live as if it weren't true, or as if it allowed exceptions. Impermanence is like the law of gravity, which operates on us whether we like it or not.

Again, the seventh Dalai Lama wrote a poem on this subject, about men going into battle.

> Spirits were high with expectations this morning,
> As the men discussed subduing the enemies and
> protecting the land.
> Now, with night's coming, birds and dogs chew their corpses.
> Who believed that they themselves would die today?

While I was giving the talks on which this is based, an American Zen master I knew fell over dead of a heart attack in the middle of an interview. He was in his early fifties. My writing partner decided not to move but to renovate his present house largely because he loved his neighbors; in the middle of the renovations, everyone's favorite neighbor—the man they called the mayor of the street—was diagnosed with a brain tumor, and within a month he was dead.

Everyone has stories like these. Just look at today's obituaries. Many of these people were elderly; many had been ill. But how many really expected they would die when they did? We hear of such things happening to other people and think it will never happen to us, but chances are that they will, one way or another. It is often true that when death finally comes, it is not expected.

5. There are many causes of death.

It seems to be a peculiarly modern problem that we think we can find a cure for everything, solve any problem. We licked polio; we eliminated smallpox; we don't have thousands in sanitariums with TB anymore; and now we want to cure everything else. We put tremendous time and energy into seeking cures for AIDS and for various kinds of cancer, and of course these are worthy projects. But we can get into the mindset where we think we're going to cure everything. We're going to eliminate death.

The fact is that we eliminate one thing and another comes up. We no longer die of consumption, but now there's AIDS. We do much better fighting some forms of cancer, but with others—despite all kinds of sophisticated treatment—we are not successful. Remissions occur, but then the cancer comes back. And we need to remember also that in large parts of the world many diseases haven't been eliminated at all. People still die from things that killed us in this country eighty or a hundred years ago but no longer do. Malaria, for instance, is still the number one killer in the world.

And that is just illness. It says nothing of war, famine, murder, suicide, car accidents, accidents of other kinds, hurricanes, avalanches, floods, earthquakes, tornadoes, and drownings. We could go on and on. If we find a way to eliminate all the illnesses we currently face, others will arise, because the earth can support only so many people, and it will take care of itself. And sooner or later the earth itself will die. It is an impermanent phenomenon like any other, with a beginning, middle and end.

To be alive, then, is to be subject to any number of causes and conditions, some of which come upon us unexpectedly and have unexpected results. To feel protected from these things is to be living in a fool's paradise. We have just been temporarily spared.

As Nagarjuna said [in Jeffrey Hopkins's translation], "We maintain our life in the midst of thousands of conditions that threaten death. Our life force abides like a candle flame in the breeze. The candle flame of our life is easily extinguished by the winds of death that blow from all directions."

At about this point in the contemplations, we begin to feel that the whole thing is senseless, that these contemplations are the concoction of a wicked and morbid imagination and that if we listen to them anymore we'll be too depressed even to live. So it is good to pause here with a word of warning: Of course this view of things is morbid and depressing, overwhelming when presented all at once, and of course there are many wonderful things in life. The fact that life is impermanent and uncertain does not mean that it is worthless. Seen correctly, these facts make life more precious. They show us that every moment is a gift.

The point of these contemplations is to correct an imbalance. We all live, too often, as if these facts of life don't exist. These contemplations on death are intended to wake us up. They awaken us ultimately to the joy and beauty of a life free of craving and grasping, a life where we see through the illusion of being young and healthy forever and drop it.

6. The human body is fragile.

I had an uncle who died at the age of twenty-two. He was slicing vegetables with a rusty knife and accidently cut himself. Within a few days he was dead.

A son of President Warren Harding apparently died because he neglected a blister and got blood poisoning. In North Carolina this summer, a huge hulking football player in wonderful physical condition—a star of the team and president of the senior class—got overheated during practice despite many precautions by his coaches. His body temperature went up to 107 degrees and the medical emergency workers couldn't get it down. He died soon after he got to the hospital.

So on the one hand the human body is enormously resilient. We have all heard stories of people who endure tremendous hardships during wars or natural diseases, or who are old and sick and seem to hang on forever. On the other hand, the body is terribly vulnerable. A microbe can kill it. A hard blow to a fragile organ can. A cut to a key artery can. Death can come quickly.

The import of all three of the contemplations in this category is the same. It isn't to scare us, though fear may come up. It isn't just to make us more careful, though it may help us take our days less for granted.

The point is that we all tend to see life following a certain pattern. We imagine youth, a long period of childhood, and a serene old age, at the end of which we peacefully expire.

That is just an idea. It is an image. Death isn't waiting for us at the end of a long road; it is with us every minute. Our lives are impermanent and fragile, our fate uncertain. The intention of these contemplations is to make that fact vivid, to call it up before us and make us see things as they really are. Whichever contemplation does that best is the one to use.

Only the Practice of Dharma Can Help Us at the Time of Death

7. Our wealth cannot help us.

The last set of contemplations is an extremely rich one for Dharma practitioners. It is in some ways a minute examination of the fourth contemplation from our earlier group: "I will grow different, separate from all that is dear and appealing to me." It can be an extremely effective, if difficult, set of exercises.

What I would encourage you to do is actually picture yourself on your deathbed. Settle into a period of meditation, establish some samadhi, then do visualization. Imagine yourself in your room, with a clear mind, waiting for the moment of death. Imagine what you might be thinking and feeling.

Wealth is a kind of shorthand in this first contemplation. Few of us think of ourselves as wealthy (though the fact is that, compared with most people from the past and in the rest of the world, we live in almost unimaginable luxury), but we all have things, we probably all have some cherished things, and we might have spent a lifetime working to accumulate them. Our book collection. Our record or CD collection. A beloved musical instrument. Our car. Our clothes. Our house. Think of all we have done to acquire the objects, especially those that we craved for a long time.

I'm not saying that there is anything wrong with such possessions. But none of them can help you at the moment of death. Pick up your favorite book, your musical instrument, your suit or dress. Your statue of the Buddha. You will have to give them all up and will never see or touch any of them again. Those objects can't ward off death or make the experience more manageable.

If that is the true reality of life and death, and if Dharma practice could be of some help to you—as it is certainly my feeling that it could—wouldn't it have been better to give more of your time to practice and less to accumulating objects that are going to turn to dust in your hands?

Tara Tulku Rinpoche pointed out to me that Americans—who pride themselves on being shrewd, hard-nosed businessmen—are actually bad businessmen. They're not watching the true bottom line at all. They are putting all of their energy into something ephemeral and ultimately unfulfilling. Even your good name, your spotless reputation, all your accumulated learning, your prizes and awards, your tenured position will not accompany you where you're going now. Why did you spend so much time earning them?

One can't help thinking of the wealthy young man in the Bible who approached Jesus. He asked what he could do to find eternal life. And Jesus—clearly seeing what was holding this particular person back—said, "Give up all that you have and follow me." The young man walked sorrowfully away. He couldn't bring himself to do that. But sooner or later we will all have to do it. It is just a matter of time. We are clinging to things that cannot last.

Krishnamurti delivered this message quite clearly. The reason that death is so hard for you is that your life has been about attachment and accumulation. "Do you want to know how to die?" he said. "Think of the thing you treasure the most and drop it. That is death."

> Avoid works of little consequence;
> And seek the path to spiritual joy,

> The things of this life quickly fade;
> Cultivate that which benefits eternally.
> —Dul Zhug Ling

8. Our loved ones cannot help.

This contemplation is the most difficult one for many people. We can see that our book collection, our music, our good reputation and our titles, our position in the community, all might have some ego in them. It might be that our devotion to them is slightly misguided. But we think our human relationships are not tainted in that way. Our relationship to our spouse or partner. Our parents. Our children. Brothers and sisters. Close friends. Our spiritual teachers. We believe we have some relationships that have a certain purity to them.

That may be true. But it is also true that our friends cannot help us when we die. They may be there (and they may not; we don't know how that will go). They may comfort us. But in the end we have to say goodbye to them and not see them again. We have to die alone. As Shantideva said [in Stephen Batchelor's translation]:

> While I am lying in bed, although surrounded by all my friends and relatives, the feeling of my life being severed will be experienced by me alone. When I am seized by the messengers of the Lord of Death, what benefits will my friends afford? What help can my relatives be? At that time the sole thing that will provide me with a safe direction will be the degree of purity in my mind-stream. But have I ever really committed myself wholeheartedly to such cultivation?

I don't know of any visualization that can make the truth of death more real to me. Picture lying in your deathbed. Imagine the person you love most in the world coming to your side. Then imagine saying goodbye to that person forever.

That is the reality of death. For most people, it is the most difficult part.

It is only natural to turn to those we love at the time of death. But despite our close bond with those people, we must finally be alone. Strong attachments only make matters worse; our departure will be marked with torment. Grasping and peace don't go together. We come into the world alone and must leave it alone.

9. Our own body cannot help.

We are really getting close to home. We have just said goodbye to the person who is nearest and dearest to us. Now we must say goodbye to our body.

Throughout our lives our body has been our closest companion. At times it has seemed to be who we are. We have spent hours washing and cleaning and clipping and oiling and combing and brushing, taking care of our body in all kinds of ways. We have fed it and rested it. We might have had differing attitudes toward it, sometimes loving it and sometimes hating it. But now this closest companion, who has gone through everything with us, will no longer be here. It will no longer take in oxygen. It will not circulate blood. This body that for so many years was so full of vitality will be lifeless. It will be a corpse.

The first Panchen Lama says it well: "The body that we have cherished for so long cheats us at the time when we need it most."

It is also true that this is not the last change that it will undergo. As a physical phenomenon the dead body, if not cremated, will decompose, and it is common in Buddhist practice to consider the stages of change and decay in order to bring the reality of death home.

Buddhist monks sometimes actually visit the charnel grounds to contemplate these other forms, to see our final fate, and there is a whole series of charnel ground meditations as well. The Mahasatipatthana Sutra, the Buddha's main teaching on what to be mindful of in meditation, offers some guidelines as to how to practice with dead bodies at various stages of decomposition. For our purposes, visualization of these stages is more practical.

As with earlier contemplations, we first calm the mind with breath awareness; then through words and visualizations we create each stage and contemplate it. It is important to make a connection between the image and our own body. One traditional formulation is "Truly, my body is of the same nature as the body being visualized. It won't go beyond this nature. It is of the same lawfulness." Our bodies don't belong to us but to nature. And nothing in nature has a stable form.

Reflecting in this way helps us come to terms with the nature of the body. We view it with wisdom, see that it can't be any other way. If fear or resistance comes up, we see that too with nonjudgmental awareness, watching it arise and pass away.

Ajaan Suwat taught me a version of this practice that I found extremely helpful. In his approach, you would start out by visualizing an inner organ of the body that you can easily picture, then watch what happens to it after death as the body goes through its stages of decomposition. When you reach the ninth contemplation (listed below)—when everything is ashes and dust—visualize it re-forming to its starting point. Finally—and I found this crucial—focus on the mind that is aware of all this. See that it is completely separate. This understanding keeps the charnel ground contemplation from becoming overwhelmingly depressing.

Both of my parents instructed me to have them cremated when they died. My father died first, and I placed his picture and the urn with his ashes on the home altar where I meditate each day. In addition to my daily Vipassana practice, I would find some time in most sittings to look at his picture and remind myself that the urn contains all that was left of his body and that I was not exempt from the same process. Such reflections sometimes aroused a powerful sense of how unstable my body is.

As I write these words, my mother's ashes now rest in an urn on the same altar. I am carrying out the same practice with her, and it is proving to be equally rich. Such teaching is the last gift that my extraordinarily generous parents were able to give me.

Charnel Ground Meditations from the Mahasatipatthana Sutra [adapted from U Silananda's The Four Foundations of Mindfulness]

1. I see my body, dead for a few days, bloated, blue, festering.
2. I see my dead body infested with worms and flies.
3. I see that all that is left of my body is a skeleton with some flesh and blood still clinging to it.
4. I further consider my skeletal corpse without any flesh, yet still spotted with blood and held together with tendons.
5. All that is left of my dead body is a skeleton with no blood stains, held together by tendons.
6. I see that now all that is left is a collection of scattered bones. The bones of the feet have gone one way, the bones of the hand another. The thigh bones, pelvis, spinal vertebrae, jaw, teeth, and skull have all come apart in different directions. They are all now just bare bones.
7. All that is left is a collection of bleached bones.
8. A year passes and I see that my dead body is reduced to being a pile of old bones.
9. These bones decay and become dust; blown apart and scattered by the wind, they cannot even be called bones anymore.

As with many deep truths, people tend to look at the death awareness meditations and say, "Yes, I know all of that. I know I'm going to die someday. I know I can't take it with me. I know my body will be dust."

And as with other things—as with the law of impermanence itself—I would say we know it and we don't know it. We know it in our heads but we haven't taken it into our hearts. We haven't let it penetrate the marrow of our bones. If we had, I can't help thinking we would live differently. Our whole lives would be different. The planet would be different as well.

If we really faced our fear of death—and these contemplations will bring it up again and again—our lives would ultimately be lighter and more joyful. I don't propose death awareness to depress us. It enhances our ability to live more fully.

If we understood the reality of death, we would treat each other differently. Carlos Castaneda was once asked how we could make our lives more spiritual, and he said: "Just remember that everyone you encounter today, everyone you see, will someday die." He's right. That knowledge changes our whole relationship to people.

During death awareness practice groups that I've led in Cambridge, I have asked people to leave the building after lunch, to walk around town, and to know that everyone they see will die; everyone is their brother or sister in death. It is a wonderful thing to do, especially after a period of death awareness meditation. It gives you a whole new attitude toward people you encounter.

Finally, life is a great teacher and death is a great teacher. Death is all around us, everywhere. For the most part—following the lead of our culture—we avoid it. But if we do open our hearts to this fact of our lives, it can be a great help to us. It can teach us how to live.

21 The Last Kiss

Fernando Kogen Kawai

Someone asked me once what it takes to do this job well. More than anything else, I think, it is the ability to enter deeply into the pain, suffering, and sadness that are a part of living and dying, and then emerge on the other side into peace and joy. Over and over again.
—James L. Hallenbeck, *Palliative Care Perspectives*

At ninety-one, Sylvia was dying in the hospital with lung cancer and end-stage heart failure. There she was, connected to the uncomfortable BIPAP pressure mask that was pushing air into her face, her hands tied to the bed in order to prevent her from taking the mask off. The doctors from the primary team understood that she could die at any moment but were very reluctant to give her any morphine to relieve her pain and shortness of breath, concerned that it could cause further respiratory depression and a possible drop in blood pressure.

It was a busy day and we had twenty-two seriously ill patients on our list, each one with complex clinical and psychosocial problems. I took a deep breath before walking into the room. After a brief contemplative pause, I brought myself to the moment and focused my attention on Sylvia. I introduced myself and asked what her understanding of the current situation was. Sylvia was remarkably awake and able to answer Yes/No questions by speaking and nodding through the mask. I listened carefully as she acknowledged her terminal condition, confirmed that she would like a Do-Not-Resuscitate/Do-Not-Intubate (DNR/

DNI) order, and asked to be disconnected from the BIPAP machine. I explained that if we were to do so she could die within a few hours, maybe a couple of days at best. She said that she understood and still wanted the mask off. I promised to give medications to palliate her pain and shortness of breath and make sure that she would be comfortable during the process. I also mentioned that I needed to speak to her husband before proceeding. "Go ahead," she said, "But please take this horrible mask off me AS SOON AS POSSIBLE!"

I knew that legally and ethically I could go ahead with liberating Sylvia from the machines. The US Supreme Court supports an individual's right to discontinue life-prolonging measures that cause pain and discomfort even if death may be an unintended consequence. That being said, I had learned from prior experiences that the patient may be ready to let go, while the wife or husband often may not. This is important because the partner becomes the decision-making surrogate once the patient loses consciousness. If the husband showed up after Sylvia got disconnected and said, "Please reconnect her," we would be in a difficult ethical and legal conflict. I have had similar cases in the past—the son of one of my former patients with advanced dementia entered into a legal fight to change his mother's living will in court so that he could proceed with a feeding tube placement. He was a lawyer who was having a hard time accepting the impending death of his mother. He did not see his mother as "terminal," and considered that withholding artificial nutrition would be "killing" her.

I took a deep breath to bring myself to the moment and focus on the communication task at hand, then called her husband, a retired psychology professor in his mid-nineties, who had a terrible cold and coughed loudly over the phone. I asked what his understanding of his wife's current condition was, and he acknowledged that she was in a terminal condition with lung cancer, severe pneumonia, and breathing problems. He also knew about her DNR/DNI status, the pressure mask, and how uncomfortable it was for her.

"I am afraid that I have some bad news," I began, and paused to allow silence in order to give him time to prepare himself.

"Please go ahead, doctor."

"Professor, your wife asked me to liberate her from the pressure mask. She feels very claustrophobic and uncomfortable with it, and mentioned that the mask is just prolonging her suffering. She understands that the mask is keeping her alive but said, 'There is no point in continuing this if there is no quality of life.' She has full understanding of her condition, and her wishes are very clear." I paused there, allowing him to process the difficult news. Often patients and families get overwhelmed with the disclosure of a bad diagnosis and prognosis. Using silence is a very powerful tool. Silence also allows time for me to focus on the nonverbal and return to my breath and body.

I knew from experience that "quantity versus quality of life" is a relatively easy concept to grasp, as opposed to focusing on the technical medical issues and numbers. I have heard inexperienced providers spend lots of time explaining that "oxygen saturation and white blood cell counts are getting better" while completing ignoring the sad fact that the patient is dying. Yes, the BIPAP machine improved Sylvia's oxygen saturation, but did it really help her? The cancer was progressing, and no machines would stop it. Right speech can make a big difference. I deliberately chose the words "Liberation from the pressure mask" instead of "withdrawal of care" and said that we would do "Everything possible to make sure that she was comfortable" rather than "there is nothing else that can be done." I also described the DNR/DNI order as "allow a natural death and not connect her to machines" instead of asking the vague question "Should we do everything in case she stops breathing and her heart stops?"

The professor carefully listened as I described the options that we had in his wife's case. "Doctor, how long will she last if we disconnect her?" he asked.

I paused and then said, "Unfortunately, her health is deteriorating quickly. She could pass within hours, possibly days. I am sorry about the bad news."

He didn't respond right away, so I asked, "How are you doing?"

Listening is one of the main palliative care procedures, and likely one of the most important things that contemplative care providers can offer their patients. I actively listened as he told me that they had been married for fifty-five years and that he was very upset with the thought of her imminent death. I tried to explain that I understood that this was shocking news and how hard this must be for him, but that the right thing to do was to respect her wishes. I knew from prior experiences that bringing the patient's wishes to the conversation is a very important part of any end-of-life discussion. The professor understood that both the medical team and the family had the ethical obligation to honor the patient's decision.

"Doctor, thank you for your time. Sylvia told me many times in the past that she did not want to suffer. I agree that we should respect her wishes. Please go ahead and disconnect her. I have a cold . . . is it okay if I come?"

"If you have the energy, I encourage you to do so," I answered. "She is so sick that a viral exposure is not going to make any significant difference at this time, and I am sure that she would like to see you."

As soon as I ended the phone conversation with the professor, I took a deep breath and paused. By now, I had been able to clarify Sylvia's goals of care (to be comfortable and to be disconnected from the machine) and had been able to update her husband, who readily agreed with the plan. The next step was for me to get the support of her primary care doctor. Many times I have seen the family leaning toward comfort care, only to have the oncologist or primary doctor show up and suggest that "maybe we could do one extra chemo or one more procedure to see if it helps." Families find it difficult to turn this option down once it's been offered, often causing the patient to go through unnecessary suffering and pain without changing the unavoidable conclusion.

I once had a case in which the family had consented for the ventilator to be removed, but the plan changed after the primary doctor said that it was "too early to give up" and that "the patient could get better." I knew I had to make sure that Sylvia's doctor was in agreement with the comfort-care treatment that we were planning. I called Sylvia's primary physician and asked what his understanding was of Sylvia's case.

He shared with me that he had taken care of her for many years and was saddened to witness her decline and deterioration. He mentioned that he had tried all treatments available but was frustrated with the results. After I explained her wishes, he agreed with the plan.

Doctors are human, and we often get attached to our patients. I had a case in which a patient with terminal liver cancer and cirrhosis signed a DNR/DNI order, saying that he did not want to prolong his suffering by being connected to machines. His hepatologist who had taken care of him for many years ripped the DNR/DNI order from the chart when he saw it and mentioned angrily that he should not "give up" and "should fight to live." When I came to follow up the next day, the patient told me, "Doctor, please forgive my doctor. He is having a hard time accepting that I am getting close to the end and will die soon." Palliative care often involves counseling of the patient, counseling of the family, *and* counseling of the primary team. After all, doctors go into medicine with the intent to save people, not to allow their patients to die. It is not unusual for doctors to experience a sense of failure that can cloud their judgment when their patients are dying.

In the meantime, Jane, our nurse clinical coordinator, was synchronizing the respiratory, nursing, and medical teams to prepare adequate morphine doses at the bedside and get everything ready. The intent was to try to keep Sylvia awake but comfortable during the "liberation from mask" procedure. Jane spoke to the nursing staff about nonverbal signs of pain, treatment, and monitoring shortness of breath. She also addressed the concerns that some staff had about opioids; we had a prior case in which a nurse became traumatized when a terminal patient died after she administered morphine to relieve his pain. Jane explained to the nursing staff that we would be starting at low doses and would increase incrementally as needed. She also mentioned that since our intent was to relieve the documented shortness of breath and pain, we were legally and ethically allowed to administer opioids. The US Supreme Court authorizes healthcare providers to administer potentially lethal doses of opioids to relieve pain even if death is an unintended consequence, as long as there is careful documentation and adequate medical adjusting of the dose based on the symptoms. These measures are very different from euthanasia, where the intent of the medical team is to kill the patient.

Other family members were also calling on the phone, and Jane calmly explained the plan to liberate Sylvia from the mask while focusing on her comfort. We knew that it was important for the family to be informed of the plan so that we could support both Sylvia and the professor in their decision, while also giving loved ones the final chance to visit with Sylvia and say goodbye.

As the phone calls continued coming in, my own anxiety and stress increased. I was pleased that we were making progress, but I was also worried about the patients that we still had to see later that day. As I felt the anxiety rising, I took deep breaths and tried to come back to the present by connecting to my body, becoming aware of the dry cough and reflux feeling in my chest as I worried about falling behind schedule. I took a deep breath in and held it. "It is what it is," I told myself. "Worrying is not going to help me take care of Sylvia or the other patients that are waiting. Better to do one thing at a time. *Now* is the time to concentrate on her—later I will see the other patients." Just a few breaths were enough to give adequate space to the worry and stress. A few more breaths, and my mind slowly quieted, letting go of all the other things that needed to get done later that day and allowing me to focus on what needed to be done right there in that moment.

It's not hard for patients and families to notice when the healthcare provider's mind is "elsewhere." If we want to provide adequate and compassionate care, the full presence of the provider is essential. Yes, the care provider and the patient will get distracted, and their minds will wander off. The practice is to bring awareness back to the patient and what is happening in the present moment—over and over and over again.

The nurse was finally ready to give Sylvia the medication, and we untied her hands and took off the mask. She immediately thanked us. As we were liberating her from the machine, her elderly husband arrived, walking cane at his side and cold mask on his face.

"Darling, we don't have much time," she said to him. "It's going to be soon."

He took off his mask. "I know," he said, and tenderly kissed her lips. He then put the cold mask back on his face and sat quietly at the bedside, just holding her hands.

As I witnessed their kiss and silent hand-holding, tears came to my eyes. I was surprised—it is a very rare event for me to cry while taking care of patients. It was a sad moment, and I felt that sadness. But I was also feeling what a privilege it was to bear witness to such an intimate moment. There was so much beauty in that kiss. I felt very connected to both of them. I felt peace while seeing Sylvia coming to terms with her mortality and accepting her end, and I felt the love of the professor in his willingness to let go of attachment and agree to respect her wishes, kissing her farewell.

Sylvia died two days later. Instead of being connected to machines and having her hands tied, she chose to rest peacefully holding the hands of her beloved husband. The tenderness of their last kiss is still present and lives on in my heart. Moments like these help me to carry on through the many challenging moments that come with being a doctor. Experiences like these help me to keep my heart open and remain connected to my patients as human beings, not just diseases and possible methods of treatment. As a palliative care provider, I often stand on the bridge between life and death, and it is my role to serve my patients and their families while they cross the troubled waters of serious illness. If I can stay present, actively listen, communicate with compassion, and accept the outcome, I hopefully will be able to effectively help the seriously ill without burning out myself.

Thank you, Sylvia. And thank you, professor.

Attunement: Meditations on Compassion 22

Frank Ostaseski

What Suffering Can Teach Us

I didn't get into this work because I was noble. I got into the work of service as an effort to try to avoid my own suffering. And perhaps that's true for a lot of us who have done some sort of service work, particularly those of us working in healthcare. I tried just about everything I could imagine to keep suffering at arm's length, but it kept encroaching. Sooner or later we stop and we turn toward the suffering. Then we learn what it has to teach us. We come to understand that suffering gives rise to compassion.

Attunement

Compassion is the capacity in each of us that enables us to be sensitive to suffering. The presence of compassion can be known not only in the heart and mind but also as an experience of the body. We sense suffering and our compassionate wish to come close to it. We can know compassion as a form of intimacy. One way that intimacy is expressed is as *attunement.*

Compassion is an attunement to exactly where the other person is, to what matters most in the moment, to the exact face of their suffering. It has no agenda, no judgments, no shoulds. We cannot help a person if we are trying to change them. I don't think we serve a person by taking them away from themselves or their suffering.

Compassion is both fierce and kind. Its fierceness allows us to approach and accept suffering when we would otherwise wish to turn away. Its kindness encourages the soul, the heart, to relax. Without the presence of acceptance and compassion we cannot open to our pain. The heart and soul won't open in the face of judgment or someone else's agenda.

What normally passes for compassion is kind words or attempts to remove the difficult circumstances that may be contributing to suffering. But compassion is not just an emotional state; it has a fierceness that actually allows us to stay present and tender; it is relational; it is a warm hand-to-hand connection. A common misunderstanding of compassion is that you should help someone to feel safe, help them feel there is *no danger.* This is fine of course if you can do it . . . but I work with the dying, and most of the time dying does not feel safe.

When compassion is present the attunement is so clear to the other or to our own hearts that we feel our selves coming closer . . . like a "soul to soul" meeting. I have found that when I am really present, grounded in compassion, the other person senses this and begins to trust and open — not because there is no danger . . . but because there is genuine understanding and companionship that is felt as support and encouragement to go toward the suffering.

It's important for caregivers to understand something about the presence of compassion: When compassion is really present, a great deal of pain and suffering may show up in your life. That is because the pain wants to expose itself to the healing agent of loving-kindness.

Steven and Rick

Some years ago, when I was guiding the Zen Hospice Project, there were two men in the house, both of whom were living with and dying of AIDS. One of them, Rick, in addition to his AIDS diagnosis had suffered a stroke. Because of that stroke and his aphasia he had trouble articulating what he wanted to say. Frustration and anger followed; it was very difficult to be with him. All of our attempts to help bounced off a sort of defensive shield that he had constructed.

Down the hall was Steven. When you went into Steven's room you felt like you were going into a sanctuary. He was almost transparent. He was very close to dying.

I went to Rick one afternoon and I said, "It looks like Steven might be dying soon, and if you want to say goodbye to him now might be the time." I helped him down the hall—he was paralyzed on one side. I eased him into Steven's room and he sat down on the bed next to Steven. I didn't say anything. I just backed out of the room and stayed in the doorway so I could just watch them a little bit. It was so beautiful. I don't think they said a word for about twenty minutes. They accompanied each other. Not trying to make anything happen, not trying to resolve anything. And after a while Rick just nodded and Steven said, "Yeah, that was great!" Rick got up and went to his room. Steven died later that afternoon.

Rick was looking at his destiny. He knew he too would be dying soon. And Steven just mirrored back to him the capacity that lives in each of us for compassion. He could sense where Rick was; he didn't need to say anything. And Rick's heart and soul just opened to Steven. Steven had simply rested in his being because he wasn't afraid to embrace the suffering—he was willing to sense suffering and be with Rick in that way.

Michael

A good friend of mine died a few months ago, someone I worked with for maybe fifteen years. One afternoon he was coming back from the hospital—he had had a bad episode and had been in the intensive care unit—and he said, "Frank, I'm not going back, that's it." I asked why? He said, "All the work we've done, I imagined I wouldn't be scared, but I'm really scared." I sat with him in silence. After a while I said, "Michael, that part of you that's scared is never going to go away. We need to find a part of you that can be with that fear. If you are aware of the fear, that means that there is a part of you that is not afraid. You don't need to get rid of the fear. You can orient to that awareness that is not afraid. You can be with your fear without being lost in reactivity to it." He looked at me and said, "That's the most comforting thing anybody's ever told me."

Being with Our Wounds

When I was a little kid, I cut my hand and ran into the house to my mother, screaming and bleeding all over the place. And she did the most miraculous thing. She wasn't always adept at these things, but this time she was really good. She grabbed the magic towel. Our magic towel was always in a place of honor—it was on the bar of the stove. She took the magic towel, she wrapped my hand up in it, she took me onto her lap, and she just embraced me. She just rocked me. And I cried and cried and cried. I was really scared. Through the presence of her touch and her not being scared of my pain, I gradually calmed down.

After I'd calmed down a bit, she said, "Let's look." And she unwrapped the towel, and she showed me the wound. She showed me that it was possible to look into our wounds and be with our wounds, that all of us can do this, that even a child can do this. It was a beautiful experience to have as a child, and it's been a great teaching in my life.

Seeing the Causes

True compassion is the capacity in each of us to stay with suffering. Compassion is not about removing suffering but about cultivating the capacity to be *with* suffering. Once we can be with the suffering, we can stop fighting it, and our defenses can fall down. And then we can see in an unobstructed way. We can see the causes of the suffering, and seeing the causes allows us to maybe do all sorts of skillful things. But we won't be able to see the causes—see what's really going on—until the defenses are down.

Doing Your Homework

Compassion requires that we get in touch with what hurts. Pain is what invites compassion to manifest. This is intimate work. We cannot do it from a distance.

If someone says to you, "I'm afraid," and you haven't really understood for yourself what it's like to be afraid—What happens to your tongue and what happens in your chest and in your big toe? What about your thoughts? Are they planning thoughts or remembering thoughts?—if you haven't done your homework, when you say, "I understand," those you are caring for will sniff out your sentimentality and your insincerity, and they'll yell out, "Bullshit!"

Important Strangers

Compassion is that aspect of our nature, a facet of our capacity to love, that arises as openness—a guidance in our work when suffering is present. One has to listen very, very carefully. Not just for the content but for the heart of the experience, listening with one's whole body.

Contemplative support means facing the truth directly. Staying in the room when the going gets rough. Allowing yourself to be really intimate with important strangers.

Turtle, Swan

Mark Doty

Because the road to our house
is a back road, meadowlands punctuated
by gravel quarry and lumberyard,
there are unexpected travelers
some nights on our way home from work.
Once, on the lawn of the Tool

and Die Company, a swan;
the word doesn't convey the shock
of the thing, white architecture
rippling like a pond's rain-pocked skin,
beak lifting to hiss at my approach.
Magisterial, set down in elegant authority,

he let us know exactly how close we might come.
After a week of long rains
that filled the marsh until it poured
across the road to make in low woods
a new heaven for toads,
a snapping turtle lumbered down the center

of the asphalt like an ambulatory helmet.
His long tail dragged, blunt head jutting out
of the lapidary prehistoric sleep of shell.
We'd have lifted him from the road
but thought he might bend his long neck back
to snap. I tried herding him; he rushed,

though we didn't think those blocky legs
could hurry—then ambled back
to the center of the road, a target
for kids who'd delight in the crush
of something slow with the look
of primeval invulnerability. He turned

the blunt spear point of his jaws,
puffing his undermouth like a bullfrog,
and snapped at your shoe,
vising a beakful of—thank God—
leather. You had to shake him loose. We left him
to his own devices, talked on the way home

of what must lead him to new marsh
or old home ground. The next day you saw,
one town over, remains of shell
in front of the little liquor store. I argued
it was too far from where we'd seen him,
too small to be his . . . though who could tell

what the day's heat might have taken
from his body. For days he became a stain,
a blotch that could have been merely
oil. I did not want to believe that
was what we saw alive in the firm center
of his authority and right

to walk the center of the road,
head up like a missionary moving certainly
into the country of his hopes.
In the movies in this small town
I stopped for popcorn while you went ahead
to claim seats. When I entered the cool dark

I saw straight couples everywhere,
no single silhouette who might be you.
I walked those two aisles too small
to lose anyone and thought of a book
I read in seventh grade, "Stranger Than Science,"
in which a man simply walked away,

at a picnic, and was,
in the act of striding forward
to examine a flower, gone.
By the time the previews ended
I was nearly in tears—then realized
the head of one-half the couple in the first row

was only your leather jacket propped in the seat
that would be mine. I don't think I remember
anything of the first half of the movie.
I don't know what happened to the swan. I read
every week of some man's lover showing
the first symptoms, the night sweat

or casual flu, and then the wasting begins
and the disappearance a day at a time.
I don't know what happened to the swan;
I don't know if the stain on the street
was our turtle or some other. I don't know
where these things we meet and know briefly,

as well as we can or they will let us,
go. I only know that I do not want you
—you with your white and muscular wings
that rise and ripple beneath or above me,
your magnificent neck, eyes the deep mottled autumnal colors
of polished tortoise—I do not want you ever to die.

The Embrace

Mark Doty

You weren't well or really ill yet either;
just a little tired, your handsomeness
tinged by grief or anticipation, which brought
to your face a thoughtful, deepening grace.

I didn't for a moment doubt you were dead.
I knew that to be true still, even in the dream.
You'd been out—at work maybe?—
having a good day, almost energetic.

We seemed to be moving from some old house
where we'd lived, boxes everywhere, things
in disarray: that was the story of my dream,
but even asleep I was shocked out of the narrative

by your face, the physical fact of your face:
inches from mine, smooth-shaven, loving, alert.
Why so difficult, remembering the actual look
of you? Without a photograph, without strain?

So when I saw your unguarded, reliable face,
your unmistakable gaze opening all the warmth
and clarity of you—warm brown tea—we held
each other for the time the dream allowed.

Bless you. You came back, so I could see you
once more, plainly, so I could rest against you
without thinking this happiness lessened anything,
without thinking you were alive again.

23 In the Silence of Leaving

Robert Chodo Campbell

Let us be silent, that we may hear the whispers of the gods.
—Ralph Waldo Emerson

The nurse manager on the oncology unit asked me to look in on Marcelo and his wife. Marcelo was sixty-two years old and dying of cancer. It originated in his colon and had metastasized to the spine and liver. This was the fourth time he'd been admitted to the unit, and this time he wouldn't be going home. The next stop was hospice, but his wife would not or could not entertain the idea of her husband dying.

I introduced myself to Mrs. Ruiz as Chodo, the chaplain on the unit. "Hello, Father," she said, assuming that because I was a chaplain I was a Catholic priest. I told her I was a Buddhist. "That's okay, Father," she said. "The Lord has sent you to us. Please call me Maria, and this is my husband, Marcelo. Can you please tell him he has to fight?" She gestured to her husband emphatically. "He is giving up," she said. "But I don't believe God is ready for him yet.

"I want to take him home and make him all his favorite dishes," she continued. "He's not eating any of the food they serve him here, and to be honest I wouldn't either."

I said hello to Marcelo. "Hello, Father," he replied. Maria offered me the chair next to his bed, lowering her voice. "Perhaps you can say a prayer, Father," adding again, "He's giving up and God is not ready for him yet."

I asked Marcelo if he would like me to pray for him. "Yes, maybe in a while that will be nice," he replied.

Marcelo had a gentle voice and a very heavy Puerto Rican accent. He was maybe 5'6", just slightly taller than his wife, with beautiful deep brown eyes and hair now grey but still thick and wavy. I could tell he had once been a handsome man. He was wearing the standard hospital gown, and I assumed it was Maria who had placed a set of rosary beads around his neck. A Bible and a small statue of the Virgin Mary were on the bedside table. He was listening to his wife and smiling.

"How are you doing today?" I asked, looking directly at Marcelo.

"Oh, he's doing much better, aren't you, *mi amor*?" answered Maria for him.

Marcelo smiled and nodded his head as if to say, "There's no point arguing with her."

I asked Maria how long they had been married. "Forty years, three months, two weeks, and three days," she replied, smiling with tears welling up in her eyes.

Marcelo looked at me and said, "She's a schoolteacher—very smart and good with numbers."

Maria continued, "I met Marcelo when I was nineteen. He was the most handsome man I had ever seen. Of course, I didn't let him know that, not at first."

Marcelo added, "We met at my cousin Rosa's wedding. Maria was the maid-of-honor. I knew the moment I saw her that I wanted to marry her, but I was too shy even to ask for a dance."

Maria laughed. "Rosa told me about her cousin Marcelo—how cute he was and how shy. She said he probably hasn't kissed a girl yet—a perfect gentleman. I wasn't going to let him get away. I walked straight up to him and said, 'Ask me for a dance.'"

Marcelo chuckled. "And I have not refused her anything since that day."

Maria began to cry and turned her head away, looking out the window. "*Ay dios mio*," she said. "Look at that beautiful sky."

Marcelo looked at me and winked.

Facing both of them, I asked, "So what brought you to the US and to New York?"

"Well," began Maria, "I wanted to be a schoolteacher ever since I was a little girl, and I wanted to get a good job in a decent school. My older sister was already living here and convinced me this was the place to find good employment and raise a family. We came here shortly after we got married. I will be retiring soon, and I have been teaching for thirty years. *Dios mio*, how it has changed." She turned to her husband, "Marcelo, tell Chodo what you have done for all these years."

Marcelo looked somewhat embarrassed. "I told you she was the smart one. I was never any good in school, but she went to college. I began working for UPS and have been there all this time."

Maria looked first at me then directly at her husband and said, "Marcelo Ruiz, for all these years you have not only worked at UPS—you have supported me, you have loved me unconditionally, and you have been the best thing that has ever happened to me. I am the luckiest woman in the world. And by the way, you are also one of the smartest *hombres* in *Nuevo York* and Puerto Rico."

It was now Marcelo's turn to cry.

We sat in silence for a few moments. Then Maria asked, "What do you do here in the hospital, Chodo?"

"Well," I answered, "I am one of the chaplains here. My job is to visit with patients and simply listen to their stories—to offer counsel and spiritual guidance, and sometimes to be with family members of the patients, much the same as the Catholic priest or the Jewish rabbi. However, chaplains are usually interfaith and serve patients of all religions if needed, as well as patients with no religion."

"So it's okay that you are a Buddhist and we are Catholic?" she asked.

"Yes," I said. "Absolutely. In fact, I would love to hear about your faith and what you think you are being called to do right now."

Looking at Marcelo, she said, "Oh that's an easy one. We are being tested right now by the Lord. We are being asked to put all our faith in him and to understand his will for Marcelo."

I thought carefully before asking my next question.

"You said earlier that you don't think God is ready for Marcelo. Is it possible that he is?"

"No," she replied. "He is not ready for my husband. Marcelo is going to get through this."

This was not the time to be talking about moving Marcelo to the hospice floor.

Maria was a smart woman. She understood what the doctor, the oncologist, and the nurse manager had said to her. She had been witness to her husband's slow and now rapid deterioration, but she was not yet ready to go through that door. After forty years, three months, two weeks, and three days, she wasn't ready to say goodbye. She wanted more time.

I turned to Marcelo and asked him if he was ready for that prayer. He said that he was getting tired and would love a prayer. The three of us held hands, and I prayed for the relief of Marcelo's suffering. I asked the lord to watch over Maria and to be with her and to show his love for her and Marcelo in the difficult days ahead.

The next morning I went to visit Marcelo. Maria was there and she looked exhausted. She told me she hadn't been home now for three days and hadn't slept for more than two or three hours each night. She had been sleeping in a chair next to Marcelo's bed, holding his hand and praying. Marcelo was visibly weaker, but his voice was still clear and strong.

"Good morning, Chodo. I'm glad you came by," he said.

"I wanted to see how you are today. What's new with you, Marcelo?" I said. "How's Maria treating you?"

He smiled. I think he was relieved by my lighthearted inquiry.

Then Marcelo told me his story. "I keep telling Maria I want to go home and be with my father in his garden."

Maria sighed. "Chodo, he is talking crazy from all the medicine. His father died thirty years ago," she said.

As a chaplain, I am always listening for the story beneath the story when visiting with patients. There is often much more being said than what is being verbalized in the moment. In my early days of training, my supervisor would say, "Remember, you cannot *not* tell your story."

Here was Marcelo speaking of his father in the garden. I wondered if this was the "heavenly father" he was referring to. I asked him, "What's it like in your father's garden?"

He replied, "I won't be sick when I am there. I will be happy, and I will be waiting for my darling Maria, but she does not have to rush."

"You see, Chodo?" Maria said. "He is talking like a crazy person. He needs to come home to our apartment, eat some good food, and he will get better this time."

We sat in silence for a minute or two. Then I ventured into delicate territory: "Marcelo, are you talking about your heavenly father?"

Marcelo took a deep breath and with a clear voice said, "Yes, Chodo." Then looking at Maria he said, "That's who I am talking about, *mi amor*."

Maria began to sob. She walked over to Marcelo and lay next to him on the bed. I left them to be with each other. The door was now open—perhaps Maria and Marcelo would be ready to walk toward it together.

The following morning Marcelo looked much worse. He seemed weaker and could barely speak above a whisper. Maria had again slept in the room overnight. There was something different about her this morning. She looked not only exhausted, but incredibly lonely.

"It is not getting better," she said. "They want me to make a decision about hospice. What do you think I should do, Chodo?" We were sitting next to each other at the side of the bed. She was holding my hand and Marcelo's.

I told her, "I think you should do what your heart tells you is best for your darling husband. I know that if he goes to hospice in this hospital he will be very comfortable and will get great care."

She took a deep breath. "Then will he get better and come home?" she asked.

"I don't think so," I replied.

We sat in silence for a moment that seemed like eternity, until I squeezed her hand gently and asked, "Are you ready?"

"Yes," she replied.

I asked Marcelo, "Are you ready?"

"Yes," he replied.

Maria made the sign of the cross and kissed her husband's hand. We prayed together for a smooth transition from the oncology unit to hospice, for continued relief from pain, and for God to watch over Marcelo.

I excused myself to let the nurse manager know that Mr. Ruiz and his wife were now ready for hospice.

I visited Marcelo every day for the next week. He actually began looking better now that he was no longer hooked up to all the tubes from the oncology unit.

On his last morning he was sitting in a chair at the side of his bed. He was in a private room. Jazz was playing softly on his cassette recorder. I pulled up a chair and sat facing him knee-to-knee, and we held hands.

"Where's Maria?" I asked.

"I sent her home last night to get a good night's sleep. I told her not to come back until this afternoon." His voice was soft, clear, and strong. "I want her to take care of herself," he said.

We sat there facing each other while he talked about his life as a young man in Puerto Rico. He told me again how he met Maria, the most beautiful girl in the world. How perfect they had been together all these years. "You know, I never thought she would marry me. She was from a very good family, aristocrats from Spain many generations ago. Her father was not very happy, but as you have seen, what Maria wants, Maria gets." He laughed softly. "*El amor de mi corazon.*"

He told me he was ready and began to cry at the thought of leaving Maria, but he wasn't worried for her. "She has her sister. They have lots of friends and other family members who will take care of her."

Quite suddenly he looked directly into my eyes and said, "Chodo, I'm dying."

"Yes, I know," I responded.

"I'm dying now," he said.

In the next moment he began to spit blood. Still holding on to his hand, I stood and reached for the emergency buzzer at the side of his bed. Within a minute the nurse was in the room with the attending physician. The physician saw what was happening and said, "Let's get him into bed. There's nothing we can do now."

The doctor said something about platelets and that he had thought this might happen. Marcelo was lifted onto the bed, and I took his hand and held it until his last breath. The doctor recorded the time and was about to leave the room. I asked him and the nurse to stay in the room with me while I prayed for Marcelo, followed by a minute of silence to honor this wonderful, gentle man's passing.

It was the first time I saw a doctor cry. When I bowed my head to end the silence the doctor said, "Thank you, Chodo, for asking me to stay. He was indeed a gentle man and much loved by the staff on the unit. He will be missed."

I called Maria and said she should come to the hospital. She asked if Marcelo was okay. Sensing the alarm in her voice I said that he's fine and asked when she planned to get there.

She said she had to get dressed and run some errands. "I am so behind in everything," she said.

I told her not to worry about the errands today. There would be plenty of time for that.

"You're right," she said. "I'll be there in an hour."

I did not want to tell her over the phone of Marcelo's passing. I knew she would be distraught and wasn't sure if her support team, her sister and friends, were around. Death is not an emergency.

I let the nurses know she was on her way. They cleaned Marcelo, and I combed his hair and placed his rosary beads in his hands, which I had folded across his chest.

If you have ever been in the room at the moment of someone's death, you have probably experienced the shift in energy that occurs and sometimes remains for minutes or hours afterward. I call it the Silence of the Leaving.

At 10 a.m. on a busy inpatient hospice unit, the sounds of the staff on the phone at the front desk and the occasional muffled cries from a family member in a nearby room were not loud enough to break into the mysterious silence of death. I sat with Marcelo's body for an hour wrapped in this soundlessness.

As a Zen monk I have sat many, many hours in silent meditation in the hopes of quieting the mind. There are often a multitude of sounds to contend with, not the least of which is the noise in my own head, the chatter that never stops.

On extended retreats in the still of the countryside, one can hear the crickets trilling in late afternoon and the cicadas at night. We awaken long before the songbirds in the morning and hear them singing as the sun rises. At our center on 23rd Street in Manhattan, the noise of the traffic outside is constant: buses crawling along, the whoosh of air-brakes every few yards, ambulances en route to the nearest hospital on the East Side, not to mention the never-ending cacophony of hammers and pneumatic drills heralding yet another skyscraper.

Within the silence that follows the final breath of the dying person is the certainty that something is occurring. In the nonmoving movement of air in the room one senses a deep, deep loneliness and at the same time the connectedness of everything.

> Like dew drops
> on a lotus leaf
> I vanish.
> —Senryu, died June 2, 1827

Four Stories about Seeing Around the Corner

24

Rachel Naomi Remen

I.

For the last ten years of his life, Tim's father had Alzheimer's. Despite the devoted care of Tim's mother, he had slowly deteriorated until he had become a sort of walking vegetable. He was unable to speak and was fed, clothed, and cared for as if he were a very young child. As Tim and his brother grew older, they would stay with their father for brief periods of time while their mother took care of the needs of the household. One Sunday, while she was out doing the shopping, the boys—then fifteen and seventeen—watched football as their father sat nearby in a chair. Suddenly, he slumped forward and fell to the floor. Both sons realized immediately that something was terribly wrong. His color was gray and his breath uneven and rasping. Frightened, Tim's older brother told him to call 911. Before he could respond, a voice he had not heard in ten years, a voice he could barely remember, interrupted. "Don't call 911, Tim. Tell your mother that I love her. Tell her that I am all right." And Tim's father died.

Tim, who had become a cardiologist, looked around the room at the group of doctors mesmerized by this story. "Because he died unexpectedly at home, the law required that we have an autopsy," he told us quietly. "My father's brain was almost entirely destroyed by this disease. For many years, I have asked myself, 'Who spoke?' I have never found even the slightest help from any medical textbook. I am no closer to knowing this now than I was then, but carrying this question with me reminds me of something important, something I do not want to forget. Something that is true of all my patients, true of myself, and true of every human being. There is a part in us all that cannot be measured, a part which transcends illness or even death."

II.

My given name is Rachel. I was named after my mother's mother. For the first fifty years of my life, I was called by another name, Naomi, which is my middle name. When I was in my mid-forties, my mother, then almost eighty-five, elected to have coronary bypass surgery as it was the only way that she could prolong her life. The surgery was extremely difficult and only partly successful. For days my mother lay with two dozen others in the coronary intensive care unit of one of our major hospitals. For the first week she was unconscious, peering over the edge of life, breathing through a ventilator. I was awed at the brutality of this surgery and the capacity of the body, even in great age, to endure such a major intervention.

When she finally regained consciousness, she was profoundly disoriented and often did not know who I, her only child, was. The nurses were reassuring. We see this sort of thing often, they told me. They called it "intensive care psychosis" and explained that in this environment of beeping machines and constant artificial light, elderly people with no familiar cues often go adrift. Nonetheless, I was concerned. Not only did Mom not know me, but she was hallucinating, seeing things that were not there crawling on her bed and feeling unseen water run down her back.

Although she did not seem to know my name, she spoke to me often and at length—mostly of the past and her own mother, my grandmother Rachel who died before I was born and who was regarded as a saint by all. She spoke of the many acts of kindness her mother had done without even realizing she was being kind. "Che-Sed," said my mother, using a Hebrew word that roughly translates as "loving-kindness." The shelter offered to those who had none, the encouragement and financial support that helped others, often strangers, to achieve their dreams. She spoke of her mother's humility and great learning and of the poverty and difficulty of life in the Russia of her childhood. She recalled the abuses and hatreds the family had experienced, to which many others had responded with anger, her mother only with compassion.

Days went by and my mother slowly improved physically, though her mental state remained uncertain. The nurses began correcting her when she mistook them for people from her past, insisting that the birds she saw flying and singing in the room were not there. They encouraged me to correct her as well, telling me this was the only way she might return to what was real.

I remember one visit, shortly before she left the intensive care unit. I greeted her, asking if she knew who I was. "Yes," she said with warmth. "You are my beloved child." Comforted, I turned to sit on the only chair in her room, but she stopped me. "Don't sit there." Doubtfully, I looked at the chair again. "But why not?"

"Rachel is sitting there," she said. I turned back to my mother. It was obvious that she saw something I could not see.

Despite the frown of the nurse who was adjusting my mother's I.V., I went into the hall, brought back another chair, and sat down. My mother looked at me and the empty chair next to me with great tenderness. Calling me by my given name for the first time, she introduced me to her visitor: "Rachel, this is Rachel."

My mother began to tell her mother Rachel about my childhood and how proud she was of the person I had become. Her experience of Rachel's presence was so convincing that I found myself wondering why I could not see her. It was more than a little unnerving. And very moving. Periodically she would appear to listen, and then she would tell me of my grandmother's reactions to what she had told her. At times they spoke of people I had never met: my great-grandfather and his brothers, my granduncles who were handsome men and great horsemen. "Devils," said my mother laughing and nodding her head to the empty chair. She explained to her mother why she had given me her name, her hope for my kindness of heart, and apologized for my father who had insisted I be called by my middle name, which had come from his side of our family.

Exhausted by all this conversation, my mother finally lay back on her pillows and briefly closed her eyes. When she opened them, she smiled at me and the empty chair. "I'm so glad you are both here now," she said. "One of you will take me home." Then she closed her eyes again and drifted off to sleep. It was my grandmother who took her home.

This experience, unnerving as it was at the time, seemed deeply comforting to my mother and became something I revisited again and again after she died. I had survived many years of chronic illness and physical limitation. I had been one of the few women in my class at medical school in the fifties, one of the few women on the faculty at the Stanford Medical School in the sixties. I was an expert at dealing with limitations and obstacles of various sorts. I had not overcome these many challenges through lovingkindness. Over time I came to realize that despite my successes I had perhaps lost something of importance. When I turned fifty, I began asking people to call me Rachel, my real name.

III.

Sometimes the particulars of how someone dies—the time, place, even the circumstances—may cause those left behind to wonder whether perhaps the event was accompanied by a healing of hidden patterns and personal issues, or answered for that person certain lifelong questions. Death has been referred to as the great teacher. It may be the great healer as well. The root word of education, *educare*, means to bring forth the innate wholeness of a person. So, on the deepest level, that which educates us may also heal us. In its essential nature life is both educational and healing. Often the innate wholeness underlying the personality of each of us is being evoked, clarified, and strengthened through the challenges and experiences of our lifetime. All life paths may be a movement toward the soul, in which case our death may be the final and most integrating of our life experiences.

When Thomas came to see me he was over seventy, a family practice physician who had been in solo practice for almost fifty years. Whole families, from grandparents to grandchildren, looked to him for help in their troubles, counted on his counsel, and called him their friend. He looked the part, too—gray-haired, kindly, his body as spare and gnarled as an old oak.

When we met, he had end-stage lung cancer and could no longer get around without the constant flow of oxygen through a nasal catheter. The previous month he had closed his medical practice. Until the last year he had never missed a day. An astute diagnostician, he had come because he knew he was dying. He proposed that we open a series of conversations about his life. He had done some reflecting on his own in recent years, but felt that sharing the process might be helpful in readying himself for death.

Thomas held no religious or spiritual beliefs, and he felt death to be an unqualified ending to life. Raised Catholic, he had left the church early and embraced science as a way to bring order to the chaos of life. It had not failed him. Life had intrinsic value for him, and he wished to examine and understand his own life and what it had meant.

It surprised me that a man so altruistic, compassionate, and reverent toward the life in others, this awed by the beauty of anatomy and physiology, held no religious or spiritual beliefs. Curious, I asked him about the circumstances under which he had decided to leave the church. Open and frank about other details of his long life, he was reticent in the extreme about this. He had left at sixteen over a specific event. I never found out what it was.

Thomas had been a loner all his life. Never married, his personal life was solitary almost to the point of asceticism. Yet he was a connoisseur of beauty in all its forms, a patron of the arts, poetry, theater, music, ballet, and literature. His library held over a thousand books.

Thomas's major commitment was to his medicine and his patients and their needs, hopes, and dreams. His devotion to them was absolute.

Very early in our discussions, I asked him how he saw his relationship to his patients. Looking at a small figurine of a shepherd with his flock that another patient had given me, he smiled: "Like that." We spent the next few weeks examining the nature of this relationship and what it had meant to him. The shepherd was the steward of his flock; he protected them from danger and helped them to find, nurture, and fulfill themselves. He delivered their young. He found the strays and brought them back to the others.

He told me many stories of his shepherding and the lives of his flock. We examined these stories together, sharing our thoughts and perspectives. In the telling and the reflection, he seemed to be unfolding a much deeper sense of what his life had meant to others and what he had stood for. In these discussions, he often used an odd Victorian phrase: his patients "sheltered" with him. He was their safety, their support, their friend. He was there for them—constant, vigilant, and trustworthy. We discussed the masculine principle of action and protection, the feminine principle of nurture and sustenance, and how these came together in the person of a shepherd. What emerged was a symbol of wholeness.

All the while, Thomas was becoming more and more ill, his breathing more and more labored. Eventually, I raised the issue of his personal isolation. Who did *he* shelter with? Who was the shepherd's shepherd? "No one," he said, the words holding more pain than he had expressed before. It became clear that he did not believe that there was a place of sheltering for him. Shepherd though he was professionally, personally he had become separated from the flock, a nonparticipant, a lost person. He seemed unwilling to go much further with this.

Puzzled, I asked him to make up a story about a lost lamb, and haltingly he described a lamb that had been lost for so long that he could not even remember that there was a flock. He had learned to survive by himself, to eat what was available, to hide from predators. "Does this lamb know that his shepherd is looking for him?" I asked. "No," he said. "The lamb had done something very bad, and the shepherd has forgotten him."

"As a shepherd yourself, would you look for a lost lamb who had done something bad?" I asked. He seemed puzzled. I reminded him of the young patient from the projects he had told me about, the one he had taken on as a guardian from the juvenile courts, the one who eventually went on to college. I asked him why he had gone after him and brought him home. "Why, he was one of mine," he said unhesitatingly. "Yes," I said. "He was one of yours." There was a brief silence and then Thomas changed the subject, but I saw he was deeply affected by the thought that the bond between the shepherd and his sheep might lay beyond judgment, and went far deeper than he had previously thought.

We talked of many other things over the next months, and gradually the image of the shepherd retreated to the back of my mind. We spoke of childhood and manhood and lost love and a very rich seventy years. It had been a good life.

At one point, Thomas was hospitalized, and his health continued to worsen. His oncologist had exhausted all treatment for his cancer and had begun to increase medications to ease his respiratory distress. Gradually, Thomas became too ill to come to my office, and in the fall I began to see him at his home. Hospice was called, and by the beginning of December he had become so short of breath that he could no longer speak. I sat with him and held his hand. Sometimes I would read him poetry or sing to him a little.

Somehow he kept hanging on. The hospice workers were surprised by his endurance. One of his nurses told me that she thought he was waiting for something. I thought perhaps she was right but had no idea what it could be. His brother had come from the east coast to say goodbye, and many of his patients had already visited and left cards and other expressions of their love.

On Christmas Eve I received a call from his hospice nurse. Thomas had been in a coma all day, and now he was having difficulty with his secretions. Would I come? As soon as I saw Thomas, I realized that he was dying. His breathing, always labored, had become shallow and intermittent. The nurse with him was young and seemed a little uncertain, so I invited her to stay as I talked to him. He did not respond in any way. We changed his sheets and made him more comfortable. Then we sat down together to wait. Gradually, the spaces between his breaths grew longer and longer, and after a while his breathing stopped.

The young nurse seemed relieved. She called Thomas's brother who said that he would fly out the next day. He asked that she call the funeral director Thomas had chosen, and she called him too. She called his oncologist to sign his death certificate. There seemed nothing more to do. I stood for a time at the foot of Thomas's bed, thinking about him and wishing him well. Then I left.

It was dark and had grown quite cold. Holding my keys in my pocket, I huddled into my coat and walked a little faster. I had almost reached my car when church bells throughout the city began ringing. For a moment I stopped, confused. Were they ringing for Thomas? And then I remembered. It was midnight. The Shepherd had come.

IV.

"Can you come and talk to the monthly meeting of our third-year residents?" my colleague asked me in an early morning phone call. "Any topic you like, as long as it's cutting edge." I began to laugh. "On the cutting edge of medicine or on the cutting edge of life?" I asked him. "Either," he replied. So I spoke to the gathering of young resident doctors about Medicine and Mystery.

The fifty young doctors present were superbly trained and breathtakingly competent. A few faculty had dropped by too, middle-aged, experienced practitioners or graying and respected teachers. After a brief discussion on the nature of Mystery, I asked them all to take a moment and recall an experience in their professional lives that they could not easily explain, a time when something occurred that changed them or caused them to wonder. I suggested they take a few moments to make some notes about this experience. After a surprised silence, everyone found pen and paper and began to write.

For the next two hours we shared these stories. Many had never been told before. Close to the end, an older physician told us this story. He had been twenty and studying to be an engineer when his brother became ill with leukemia. When his brother began losing his struggle to live, his parents asked him to come home from school to be with the family. Once there he had been given the job of reading to his brother.

The story he told us happened the day before his brother died. He had been sitting with him in his bedroom, reading to him. His brother lay in his bed with his eyes closed, breathing with effort. As he read he would glance up occasionally to find that his brother had not moved. He was not even sure if he was awake but, not knowing what else to do, he continued to read.

He had been reading aloud for about an hour when he felt his brother's hand on his arm. Glancing over, he saw that his brother's eyes were open and shining with excitement. He was staring at a blank wall. "Sam," his brother said. "Look! There's someone here! Someone has come! Can you see him, Sam?"

So he closed the book and looked very carefully at the wall. "I couldn't see a thing," he told us. "But I could *feel* it. There was something in the room with us, a presence—deeply loving and infinitely kind." He felt his heart drawn to it as if it were claimed. Deeply moved, he took his brother's hand.

A few silent seconds passed, and suddenly he knew with absolute certainty that he was meant to become a doctor. After his brother died, he returned to school, changed his major, and went on to study medicine. The group sat quietly waiting for more, but the doctor had nothing more to say.

After the rounds, he came up to talk a bit. Sensing that there was more to his story, I asked him about it. "Yes," he told me. "What had happened was a little different, and I felt uncomfortable speaking about it in front of the others."

"It's not that I knew that I was meant to become a doctor," he told me. "What I knew was that I *was* a doctor. I had always been a doctor. That I had been born with a doctor's soul in me. Whatever it was that came for my brother came for me, too. It felt like a sort of healing, a coming back to my true self." He stood looking thoughtful. "Perhaps it was that sort of thing for us both," he said.

Several days later, I met one of the resident doctors in the corridor who wanted to talk about the rounds a little more. During the discussion it had seemed to him that the familiar meeting room with its windowless gray walls, gray chairs, and gray carpet had become another sort of place entirely. He had been surprised that there were so many stories of Mystery among the group of physicians.

Several questions had come up for him afterward. He looked away, slightly embarrassed, but he continued on. Did I think that the practice of medicine could become a practice, like meditation or prayer? Could it bring us into a closer, deeper relationship with the Unknown?

I looked at his tired, young face struggling with a new way of seeing his work. People brushed by us in the corridor, hurrying as always. I thought of compassion, harmlessness, altruism, service, and covenant—the qualities, thousands of years old, inherent in the ancient Hippocratic Oath. They seemed to me to define a profoundly spiritual way of life. "Yes I do," I told him. "Mystery once occupied the same central place in medicine that science occupies now. Perhaps it still does."

Kindness

Naomi Shihab Nye

Before you know what kindness really is
you must lose things,
feel the future dissolve in a moment
like salt in a weakened broth.
What you held in your hand,
what you counted and carefully saved,
all this must go so you know
how desolate the landscape can be
between the regions of kindness.
How you ride and ride
thinking the bus will never stop,
the passengers eating maize and chicken
will stare out the window forever.
Before you learn the tender gravity of kindness,
you must travel where the Indian in a white poncho
lies dead by the side of the road.
You must see how this could be you,
how he too was someone
who journeyed through the night with plans
and the simple breath that kept him alive.
Before you know kindness as the deepest thing inside,
you must know sorrow as the other deepest thing.
You must wake up with sorrow.
You must speak to it till your voice
catches the thread of all sorrows
and you see the size of the cloth.

Then it is only kindness that makes sense anymore,
only kindness that ties your shoes
and sends you out into the day to mail letters and
   purchase bread,
only kindness that raises its head
from the crowd of the world to say
it is I you have been looking for,
and then goes with you everywhere
like a shadow or a friend.

Finding What Life Is

25

Shodo Harada

I am seventy now. Things are happening with my body that are clearly about aging. In Buddhism, there are these four great teachings: being born, growing old, growing sick, and dying. For all of us these are part of life, and these are what we suffer with. We send off friends to die. We feel our own bodies growing older, and we know that it is coming for us.

In the Tang dynasty in China there was a Zen master named Master Dogo. He was going to a funeral of a friend of his, and he took his student Zengen. In the house was the coffin with a dead body in it, and Zengen began hitting the side of the coffin saying, "How about it? Is this person alive or dead?" Master Dogo replied, "I'm not going to say he's alive, and I'm not going to say he's dead; I'm just not going to say."

It seems like this would be a strange question to ask, but Zengen was asking seriously about this grey area, about the point of this whole question that all of us worry about. What Zengen really wanted to ask was this: "When a living person thinks about death, and this person in the coffin's death, are they the same thing or are they different?"

A person who is alive imagining what death is like and the actuality that a dead person is manifesting are two different things. Although it seems dissatisfying that the teacher would not say he's living or dead, in fact that's a correct answer because the manifestation of that person in the coffin is not something we can know from a dualistic point of view. It is not an experience of death that is relative to an experience of being alive. If Master Dogo were to say he's alive or he's dead, he would be speaking dualistically about something that is not a dualistic experience.

Master Dogo's answer was accurate. If he were to speak about death, it could only be in relation to being alive, and a mental idea about death and dying. He's not going to speak about it in an untrue way. He also knew the state of mind of his student. Zengen was considering very deeply what it means to be alive, what it means to be totally alive, and in that comes his consideration of what it means to be dead. What is death then? In what way does being alive have to do with being dead? Master Dogo knew very well where Zengen was teetering. And so that's why he would not say, because it would only be a relative answer. Zengen was poised to know a deeper answer.

To look at this further we look at the words of Shido Munan Zenji. He was the grandfather teacher of the great Zen master Hakuin Zenji. Master Shido Munan's enlightenment poem is this: "While being still alive to die and die completely." Shido Munan Zenji is saying that we are only mentally anticipating this question of death. He is saying that instead when we are still alive we should die completely while we are alive. What this means is to throw ourselves completely into whatever it is we are doing. In this poem he's not talking about suicide. He's saying when we become what we are doing completely, we let go of this dualistic approach of living or dying. We completely become what we are doing without a dualistic sense of a doer and a doing. We give our total life to it.

The founder of the Soto sect, Master Tozan, who lived around the same time as Master Dogo, was asked by a monk, "When it is so cold and so hot, isn't there some way we can get out of that? When it's so cold to not have to be in such a cold place, and when it's hot to not be in a hot place? What way is there to get out of the pain and discomfort?" Master Tozan said, "When you're so cold, why don't you go where there is no cold? And when you're so hot why don't you go where there is no hot?" And the monk asked, "Where is this place where there is no cold nor hot?" To which Master Tozan replied, "When you are cold become completely cold. When you are hot become that hot so completely there is no longer any idea about hot or cold. When you are alive, live so totally that you don't even have an idea that you're alive, and when you die, die totally and completely. Do these things so thoroughly that there is not an idea left."

My teacher, Yamada Mumon Roshi, was from a place in the deep mountains. His father was a local politician and really wanted his son to be a lawyer, so when he was young Roshi went to Tokyo to Waseda University. But he was discontented because he had read in the *Analects of Confucius* some lines that had left him troubled and puzzled. These lines said that a true world would be one where we have no suspicions and no need of judges and lawyers. In a true world we would not even need money; we would always be supporting and helping each other in the ways that we can.

Having read this, Yamada Mumon Roshi felt that this was the actual truth. He did not want to become a lawyer; he wanted to live in a world that could be a place of no suspicion. He was dissatisfied with what he was studying. Becoming a lawyer lost all meaning for him. He lost his motivation and started to fail his classes. As the other students were progressing through school, he was reading Buddhist texts and failing one exam after the next. He had a question: How could he bring forth this world he felt was right, a world with no suspicions, a world with no lack of faith in each other?

One day in Tokyo he went to a teaching by Kawaguchi Ekai Roshi, who had been in Tibet. There he had found and brought back *The Way of the Bodhisattva* by Shantideva. The text that Ekai Roshi taught was this: If we all wanted everyone to walk comfortably on the earth we could cover the earth with leather, and it would be soft for everyone. But covering the whole earth is impossible. If we put leather under our own feet, everywhere we walk is the same as walking on an earth that is covered with soft leather. If we want to make an earth that is protected by a huge umbrella, that's impossible, but if we walk under an umbrella, we are guarded by it. If we want to liberate all the billions of people in the world, that is fairly impossible to imagine. But if we bring forth the bodhisattva vow to liberate all beings, then from every single person who has made this deep vow, it spreads exponentially to others who also want to liberate people. In this way, from one person to the next, like one candle lighting another candle, this great vow to end suffering spreads until the whole world is a sea of light.

Mumon Roshi became a disciple of Ekai Roshi. But soon Mumon Roshi became sick with tuberculosis, and in those days there was no medicine for that. The doctors said, "We can't save him; just let him do whatever he wants to now." He went back to his house in the country and was put into a room, and when the servants would come in to bring his food they would hold their breath and leave as soon as possible. Mumon Roshi began feeling like he was a danger and a burden to the people around him. "People don't want me here; I'm really just a problem." He began to feel resentful and terrible. He had failed miserably in school; then when he went to train he had gotten really sick, so sick that no one wanted to be around him. More and more he felt that there was no point in his staying alive.

It was a day in June. On this morning when he awoke he was feeling better than usual, not coughing as much, so he crawled onto the wooden porch. On that day there was a cool breeze blowing. In that cool breeze he could see the heavenly white bamboo flowers moving. He was feeling particularly good that day. Suddenly it hit him: this wind, this breeze, what is that? What is this breeze? And suddenly he realized he had all this time been given life by air. This air had always been supporting him; he had always been breathing this air without realizing it. All his friends had been passing him, he had been failing, all the servants hated him and did not want him around. But now he found out that this air—not only the air, but this great nature, and water—these things had never deserted him. Air had kept him alive, these things he had not noticed, this great all-embracing energy, without him even noticing, kept him alive to bring him to this day.

Suddenly he felt conked on the head by something heavy, and he awoke to the fact that his life was supported by everything in the universe. He directly got this. On that morning he was completely transformed by understanding these natural blessings. Water is given on this earth to us. Air comes right to us. We are given all of these natural ways of being supported for free. They are blessings that are given to us and from them we stay alive. He rediscovered his worth, his value, as simply being someone who is alive. He dropped the whole idea that he was worthless and that no one wanted him around, and he got stronger and stronger; within a month he was walking outside and doing regular work. Forty years later he had never been to see a doctor; he was living a very full life and putting all of his energy into teaching Zen to people all over the world. I was able to see this right in front of me because I was his attendant.

Once the Buddha was asking his disciples, "What is the Buddhadharma?" A disciple said, "It is the length of one day; in this one day it is as if we are born and die." Buddha said to this disciple, "You have realized the outer skin of the Buddhadharma." The next disciple said, "It is the time during one meal; during this one meal a landslide could kill someone." Buddha said, "You have realized the flesh of Buddhadharma." A disciple said, "It is only one breath." To this the Buddha said, "You have understood the marrow of Buddhadharma." In this one breath we actually live and die. In this one breath we have a sharp focus. See death clearly. Don't take your gaze away from it. But it can't be in a blurry foggy way. It has to be this direct seeing, with our precise focus, right there.

In his last poem, Masaoka Shiki wrote: "The gourd flower is blooming, the phlegm is stuck in my throat now; is this the Buddha?" He'd previously written that Zen is to be able to die anytime, anywhere, but now he realized it is to live anytime, anywhere, no matter what's happening.

In this we can see that we are missing something. We are missing a focus. To see this being-aliveness with a sharp exact focus, to really look into that and be absorbed, and to find out what that actually is. Isn't that the most important thing, to find out what life is?

Imagining People Well 26

Ira Byock

To come directly into harmony with this reality
Just simply say when doubt arises, "Not two."
In this "not two" nothing is separate,
Nothing is excluded.
—Sengcan, third Zen patriarch

The Phenomenology of Well-Being

My awakening to the shortcomings of the current, problem-based taxonomy of illness and dying came in 1978, when I encountered the phenomenon of well-being.

As a licensed physician still in training in a busy safety-net hospital in Fresno, California, I was responsible for caring for seriously ill people, some of whom were dealing with the symptoms and difficult predicaments of incurable conditions. I was called to be a doctor, to be of service, and this often made an inherently difficult job a bit easier. But every once in a while I'd meet a patient who, knowing full well that he or she was dying, described himself or herself as "well." It seemed incongruous, unexplainable within what I'd been taught and was learning.

Mr. Rodriguez's cancer had spread to his liver. He knew it and understood it meant he was dying.

"Mr. Rodriqguez, how are you today?" I asked, before inquiring specifically about his pain, his breathing, how he slept, and whether he was able to move his bowels. He looked at me and smiled. "I'm well, doctor. How are you?"

I found myself replaying that brief interaction in my mind again and again over the next few weeks. Initially, I wondered if his response was merely his deep graciousness, then worried that he might be suffering euphoric side effects from his pain relievers and medications. But what if he had chosen his words carefully? Could a person be "well" in the midst of dying?

Why did it prove nearly impossible for my colleagues and I to alleviate the suffering of some, while others, like Mr. Rodriguez, expressed a sense of well-being even while enduring significant pain? Would it be possible to make this experience of wellness available to more patients? If so, how?

As I absorbed the technical knowledge of skills in medicine, I continued to be fascinated by these questions, recognizing that within them lay answers I needed in order to become the doctor I yearned to be.

My clinical career evolved to include both emergency medicine and hospice care. Along the way I met many patients whose stories offered rich human experience for me to ponder. I learned that dying is not only about suffering and its avoidance, that some people evince a sense of well-being during their last months, weeks, days, and hours of life. This appeared clinically—and anthropologically—undeniable, but I found myself struggling to convey many people's stories through the language of medicine. In trying to explain to medical colleagues what I was observing about the personal experience of suffering of some patients and their families, and the expressed sense of well-being of others, I often found myself searching different theoretical and professional frameworks for terms and taxonomies.

The stakes were high. In the late 1970s hospice was in its infancy and rarely supported by insurance policies or governmental payers. In order to be adopted into the mainstream of healthcare, hospice needed to show a difference between the experiences of patients that died in a hospital and those who spent their last days under hospice at home. If our field was unable to name this capacity for positive experience, we would be unable to measure it. And if we couldn't measure meaningful distinctions between experienced outcomes of care, how could we refine clinical approaches?

Palliative care physicians Balfour Mount and John Scott wrote a seminal paper in *The Journal of Chronic Disease* articulating this challenge:

> I shall long remember the young patient who in dying commented that his final months (which had been characterized by relentless physical deterioration and considerable suffering) had been "the best year of my life." The day he made that comment this young athlete, scholar, and executive who had measured 10/10 on the QL throughout his life, measured 2/10. Clearly he was referring to something not embraced by the scales measuring activities of daily living and not reflected in the Spitzer QL.

Embedded within the Spitzer Quality of Life Index is an assumption that as functional capacity declines—particularly functional independence—quality of life declines. So what's the "something" not embraced therein?

Pioneering clinicians had given us theoretical frameworks for understanding suffering as a personal experience. Dame Cicely Saunders coined the term and concept of "total pain"—physical, emotion, social, and spiritual distress. Eric Cassell defined suffering as a sense of impending disintegration experienced by a person, and Viktor Frankl emphasized the felt loss of meaning and purpose as a basis for human suffering.

As valuable as these constructs and terminologies were to understanding the range and variety of patients' suffering, the opposite pole of human experience remained unencompassed. Confucius said, "The beginning of wisdom is to call things by their proper name." What, then, was the proper name for positive experience?

The Power of Stories to Expand the Realm of the Possible

Mount and Scott realized that the narratives of real people offer a corrective to the filters (or blinders) of our measures and methodologies. So I immersed myself in stories, particularly those that conveyed positive experiences of individuals with advanced illness. I began to realize that our world is bounded by our imagination. This may sound abstract, but I mean it in a most practical, tangible sense. Helen Keller wrote, "The only thing worse than being blind is having sight but no vision."

After years of alienation, harsh criticism, rejection, or frustration, two sisters were able to establish authentic appreciation for one another. A father confronted his past misdeeds and reached out to the children and previous wives he had alienated to ask for and express forgiveness, gratitude, and love. Such anecdotes, stories, and experiences stretch our imagination, expanding the realm of the possible for ourselves and those we serve.

Running through these accounts were themes of adaptation. Some people acclimatized themselves to bodily discomforts and disabilities, or found a way to absorb the emotional grief of current and coming losses and their impending death, and continued to find life worth living. Often they grieved, let go of losses, and shifted emotional energy to realms of life that remained satisfying. Remarkably, this reconfiguring of the individual's personhood seldom involved a loss of ego integrity. In fact, such people emerged with a retained or enhanced sense of meaning and purpose.

A particularly common pattern entailed a person reluctantly letting go of his professional responsibilities and aspirations as illness progressed, devoting proportionately more emotional energy and time to his friends and family. The stories are as unique as faces, but they reveal a core commonality: the things in life that matter most to people are almost always other people.

Saying the Things That Matter Most

Steve Morris was dying hard. When the hospice team met him, Steve was struggling for every breath and was unable to walk without gasping for air, yet was unable to sit still because of the anxiety that defined his life. He was scared of dying and suffered through every waking moment.

Steve had been a lineman for the phone company before a heart attack and emphysema forced his retirement. He was a real Montana cowboy—living for his horses, winning numerous riding competitions, always willing to teach horsemanship to any child eager to learn. He was a man's man, not one to express emotions or even admit to having them. Work and his horses had often come before relationships and family.

Now he was at the end of his rope. Specialists had exhausted every hope, including the lung transplant he had desperately sought. And while Steve was the one dying, he was not the only victim. His wife Dot was his constant companion, nurse, and co-sufferer. If she was out of sight for more than a minute, he would ring his bell or shout in his panicked, muffled voice, "Dot. Dot!"

It took our hospice team two weeks to gain Steve's confidence through a combination of pharmacy, counseling, and pragmatism. This included meticulous medication management; carefully selected relaxation tapes; practical suggestions for things like the placement of his recliner; and volunteers to spell Dot so she could shop for groceries, see her own doctor, and get a few moments of rest. These efforts, drawing on the experience and resources of palliative care, helped diminish—at least slightly—Steve's breathlessness and paralyzing fear.

As we learned more of Steve's personal history, we realized that his anxiety stemmed in part from the fractured nature of several key relationships and from his complex, conflicted family life. One Thursday, while I was visiting Steve and Dot at home, I told them that over the years I'd observed people often value saying four things to one another before they say goodbye:

(1) "Please forgive me."
(2) "I forgive you."
(3) "Thank you."
(4) "I love you."

I explained that the first two are because in any significant relationship there will always be some history of hurt.

"Those are really good, doc," Steve responded with unexpected enthusiasm. "Write those down for me, will ya?"

At my next scheduled home visit, Steve was sitting up, awaiting my arrival. He and Dot excitedly related the events of the past weekend. On Sunday their children and grandchildren had come over for dinner. At the table, Steve had announced he had some things he needed to say. "You know the doctors tell me that this emphysema is finally going to get me. And I know I haven't always been the best father, or husband," he paused, gathering breath and confidence. "But I love you all, and there are some things I want to say." With his eyes on my handwritten list, he recited the four things in his own words.

The effect was remarkable. Although his anxiety did not disappear in the wake of his remarks, its grip weakened. Tenderness and affection that had not been present for years, if ever, were now evident in the family's interactions. Steve's life didn't become easy, but it did become less anguished. The quality of Dot's life and their family life certainly improved.

Ironically, as he faced life's end, Steve said he was happier with himself than he could ever remember. In the process of dying, he was becoming well within himself and helping his family to become closer and more openly loving.

I realized that I had been observing a dynamic that was akin to the toddler becoming a preschooler, the young adult leaving home, the person at midlife who finds himself or herself divorced or with career uncertainty. Throughout life, crises that threaten the integrity of the person again and again offer the most opportunity for personal growth.

Marie de Hennezel observed in *Intimate Death*:

> Life has taught me three things. The first is that I cannot escape my own death or the deaths of the people I love. The second is that no human being can be reduced to what we see, or think we see. Any person is infinitely larger, and deeper, than our narrow judgments can discern. And third, he or she can never be considered to have uttered the final word on anything, is always developing, always has the power of self-fulfillment and a capacity for self-transformation through all the crises and trials of life.

Our Ability to Guide

Understanding how individuals approaching death are able to transition from experiencing a sense of meaninglessness and impending annihilation to a sense of wholeness and "wellness" has profound practical implications for psychosocial and spiritual assessments and interventions. If a sense of impending disintegration and the loss of meaning underlie suffering, it is not surprising that a sense of well-being involves a preserved—or enhanced—sense of integrity and meaning.

The assertion that "people die as they have lived" is a disservice to the very people we seek to serve. Although some people may indeed die as they lived, when construed as a prediction the statement also disserves clinicians by constraining their therapeutic imagination and narrowing the range of potential interventions. At its worst, this fatalistic attitude provides an excuse for therapeutic nihilism.

Over time I found that predictable tasks often formed the emotional, relational, and spiritual work of completing and closing a personal life. I elaborated a working set of developmental landmarks that formed the topography of the journey through terminal illness.

The process is only vaguely sequential. Individuals come to the experience of serious illness with some tasks and realms further developed than others. In most cases, however, the sense of completion of various tasks is durable and satisfying.

I think of it as starting from the outermost point—interface with our

Developmental Landmarks	**Developmental Taskwork**
Sense of completion with worldly affairs	• Transfer of fiscal, legal, and formal social responsibilities
Sense of completion in relationships with community	• Closure of multiple social relationships (employment, commerce, organizational, congregational): ▹ Expressions of regret ▹ Expressions of forgiveness ▹ Expressions and acceptance of gratitude ▹ Leave taking; saying goodbye
Sense of meaning about one's individual life	• Life review • Telling one's "stories" • Transmission of knowledge and wisdom
Experienced love of self	• Self-acknowledgment; Self-forgiveness
Experienced love of others	• Acceptance of worthiness
Sense of completion in relationships with family and friends	• Fullness of communication and closure in each of one's important relationships: ▹ expressions of regret ▹ expressions of forgiveness and acceptance ▹ expressions of gratitude and appreciation ▹ acceptance of gratitude and appreciation ▹ expressions of affection ▹ Leave-taking; saying goodbye
Acceptance of the finality of life—of one's existence as an individual	• Acknowledgment of the totality of personal loss represented by one's dying and experience of personal pain of existential loss • Expression of the depth of personal tragedy that dying represents • Decathexis (emotional withdrawal) from worldly affairs and cathexis (emotional connection) with an enduring construct • Acceptance of dependency as a normal part of life

Developmental Landmarks	Developmental Taskwork
Sense of a new self (personhood) beyond personal loss	• Self-awareness in the present
Sense of meaning about life in general	• Achieving a sense of awe • Recognition of a transcendent realm • Developing/achieving a sense of comfort with chaos
Surrender to the transcendent, to the unknown—"letting go"	In pursuit of this landmark, the doer and "taskwork" are one. Here, little remains of the ego except the volition to surrender.

physical and social environment—and working inward. Thus, a primary stage in completing a life involves attending to business and legal responsibilities. For most people this involves deeds, titles, accounts, passwords. It should include formal healthcare directives, including a durable power of attorney for healthcare. For many of us it includes wills. These are the basic safety and security tasks of social life.

Beyond these basic pragmatic tasks, people have opportunities to complete relationships (which can extend to reconciling strained relationships) and explore and achieve a sense of meaning, a sense of worth, and an unending connection to a larger whole, whether it be God, nature, family, or community. In the course of progressive illness and dying, each dimension of our being represents opportunities to grieve, complete, and celebrate.

Observed patterns of interpersonal and intrapersonal growth offer clinicians a topography for supportive counseling. The goal can then be to help patients feel complete (nothing left undone) in each realm of life so that they are able to let go of the pieces that become less relevant to their new life situation. Previously vital parts of their lives—professional roles and reputation, civic and social activities, even close personal relationships—can be released and allowed to fall away.

It is rare for someone to smile broadly and say that she is well in the hours before death. But I suspect more people do experience a sense of well-being as they withdraw more and more deeply, as the rest of us become less and less relevant to the intimate journey they are on. I believe my father was well during his final hours. I finally stopped checking because I was aware that responding to my questions was taking enormous effort, calling him back from dreamtime and work.

As the process of life completion unfolds it is common for various spheres of a person's life to become less relevant. When the person feels that nothing more needs to be done or accepts that nothing more can be done—within any given realm of activities, responsibilities, and aspirations—a natural release can occur. The person then has the opportunity to dissolve out of life, allowing the peaceful, transcendent passage that clinicians sometimes witness. But unless our language and understanding allow us to acknowledge the full breadth of human experience, our ability to guide the people we serve will be limited.

Growing Out of Life

Peter Rodis, a gifted clinical psychologist, a dedicated teacher at Dartmouth, and also a dear friend, was diagnosed with a progressive incurable cancer. His experience is powerfully expressed in a brief series of emails we exchanged during his last months of life. I share his words with his permission.

The exchange began during a time after I had not seen him for several months. I awoke one morning with Pano (as everyone called him) on my mind. I emailed him to say that I was thinking of him. Here's the response I got:

Wednesday, August 6, 2014

Dear Ira and Yvonne,

I miss you, too, and I would love to hear your voices.

As I think you know, I'm in the timeless time before the end actually

> comes. I am spiritually in a warm and gentle place. My body must pass through its sufferings every day, which are still intermittent, not constant. I can breathe, love, write, play, be with others. Some days my body feels as if it is even uplifted a bit.
>
> . . . But two and a half months ago, the prognosis given was 2–4 months. So while anything can happen at any time, I focus on keeping myself as strong and well-nourished as possible.
>
> The shock of knowing I'll die has passed. And the sorrow of it comes only at moments. Mostly, deep underneath, there is quiet, joyous anticipation and curiosity; gratitude for the days that remain; love all around. I am fortunate.
>
> Energy is very variable, but I will call soon . . .
>
> Pano

Three days later I sent another email, saying that I missed him. He replied:

> It's funny, "missing"—though a real feeling—does not have long roots these days. Instead of regret over wantings unanswered, there seems to rise instead strong impressions of presence and fulfillment, as if the things we fear lost or impossible are as realized as anything we "actually" did. Some kind of spontaneous Einsteinian reconfigurement of time, in which what might be has as much status as what (according to our senses, memories, etc.) is.
>
> . . . A surprisingly kind remaking of the phenomenologies of longing or desire, which make one feel that even if a magic genie appeared, sworn to fulfilling your every whim, you'd honesty thank him and send him back on home. Perhaps the one wish that would alter all this is if the wish to live could be granted. But the refusal of this wish is (though still so deeply unwanted) the other side of adventure, the leap that is so full of surprises.

Imagination and Empathy

The framework of human development does complement the problem-based model of medicine. But it is not enough. Particularly for those patients whose suffering persists after applying our best protocols and potions, more is required. In addition to "left brain" requirements for conceptual frameworks and language, our "right brain" capacity for imagination is needed.

Without imagination, true empathy is not possible. The difference between sympathy and empathy is a willingness and ability to imagine the experience of the other. What we can give another in these intimate processes is our presence and willingness to suffer with them. This empathic use of imagination carries risk. Some people we meet are deeply wounded, some broken in mind or spirit, some in the midst of suffering tremendous losses.

If I can somehow manage to see the world as if looking through the other's eyes, hear the person's story as if I were its teller, I can then use this imaginative alignment to explore what may still be achievable within the suffering person's hopes, values, and sources of meaning and satisfaction.

Creative Therapeutics

An informed imagination is a doctor's most powerful therapeutic tool. Without it, a doctor's care risks becoming algorithmic and devoid of creative generosity.

Confronted with a patient whose suffering persists, an impoverished ability to imagine what can be done to alleviate the person's distress can lead to a fatalistic nihilism or to the conclusion that hastening the patient's death is reasonable. On the other hand, a rich clinical imagination can make it possible to perceive—and therefore achieve—valuable events, interactions, or temporary changes in circumstances within seemingly daunting and hopeless situations.

From a stance of imaginative alignment, it is possible to stand shoulder to shoulder with the other and ask: How might this story unfold in ways that feel right? What might success look like? What can still be worth living for?

If we are able to imagine a patient becoming well—not cured, but *well* within himself or herself—it is far more likely we will be able to help the person in finding his or her own way to well-being.

Creative imagination requires sufficient self-awareness and stillness to be able to look through the eyes of the other and perceive some light ahead. The process is not only familiar and intuitive but over time can be trained and strengthened. Any doctor or counselor who has struggled to ease the distress or brighten the life of a patient has employed imagination for therapeutic intention. In the vernacular the process is often referred to as "racking my brain." That's the term I would have used during the many months I helped care for Sharon.

Sharon's Very Good Day

Sharon was just fifteen when I met her. She was suffering from cystic fibrosis. CF, as it's called, results from a genetic defect that makes the secretions of CF patients thicker than normal. Think of phlegm with the consistency of caramel. Most people with CF eventually succumb to recurrent bronchial infection and emphysema. In recent years, advances in CF treatment have led to affected people living into their 30s. Some patients receive lung transplants and live even longer.

Cystic fibrosis is a nasty disease under the best of circumstances, but Sharon's circumstances were far from the best. Her disease attacked not just her lungs, but also her digestive tract. Sluggish secretions clogged ducts carrying enzymes from her pancreas and bile from her liver. So in addition to her respiratory problems, she was undernourished. There would be no transplant for her. She'd never live to be thirty, and at least part of her knew it.

Sharon was an outwardly tough kid. As a palliative-care consultant I was asked by her pulmonologist to meet and help care for Sharon. He warned me that it would not be easy to develop a satisfying doctor-patient relationship with her. "If looks could kill, there'd be a pile of dead doctors and nurses at her door."

Whenever Sharon was admitted to the hospital—which was often and usually for two to three weeks at a time—she kept the curtains in her room drawn and the lights off, and she left strict instructions not to be disturbed as she slept through the mornings into the early afternoons. The nurses called her the princess of darkness. I came to see her tendency to "cocoon" in her room as a futile attempt to protect herself until she could magically emerge into a happier world.

Early in our relationship, I felt the daggers in her look and tone of voice. When I introduced myself to her, she said, "I know who you are. You're Dr. Death." She projected a steely exterior, but I could also see the warm, loving, hopeful interior of this frightened, angry teenage girl. I understood why "breaks my heart" was the phrase nurses and social workers frequently used when discussing Sharon and her situation.

The medical center was well over an hour drive from her home. Because of her job and family finances, Sharon's mother could only visit intermittently. During her long confinements, I stopped by the pediatric floor to visit with Sharon at the end of each day, my last task before heading home from the hospital. Sometimes I would bring along a bottle of sugarless flavored water from the gift shop, one of the only "treats" she was officially allowed. Over time, my genuine desire to befriend her—and my persistence—wore her down. Before long she accepted my visits and eventually seemed to appreciate them.

Over the months we forged a doctor-patient relationship that gradually became a doctor-patient friendship. I spent many hours in Sharon's room. I respected her right to set rules in her space and learned that some things were inviolable.

Sharon religiously watched Jeff Corwin's show on Animal Planet every weekday afternoon. If you visited Sharon during this show, you either sat down and kept quiet or left and came back after it was over. Woe to anyone—doctor, nurse, respiratory therapist, or housekeeper—who tried to interrupt.

One day in the midst of my ongoing struggles to think of something—anything—I could do to lighten Sharon's mood, it occurred to me: Jeff Corwin was a source of meaning for Sharon. Maybe he could also be a source of purpose. I suggested that she write him a letter.

Maybe she could ask to exchange letters or even to meet him. "What have you got to lose?" I said.

At first she dismissed it outright. "He'd never get it," she said. But I could tell she secretly liked the idea. "I'll make sure he receives it if you write it," I reassured her, though I had no idea at the time how I'd actually do that.

With encouragement from me and after some editing by her mother, a night nurse, and myself, here is what Sharon produced:

> Dear Jeff,
>
> I have wanted to meet you for a long time. I love to watch your shows because they brighten my day, especially when I'm in the hospital. I'm in the hospital a lot because I have cystic fibrosis and the related problems of diabetes, osteoporosis, and cirrhosis of the liver.
>
> I love all animals. I am 17. I want to learn about all of the planet's animals. I have a special love of the ocean and want to become a marine biologist. I also love snakes and want to explore becoming a herpetologist.
>
> There are also many other careers I have an interest in exploring, including being a veterinarian, but I don't want to take too much time here to write them all down.
>
> I think it's enough to say that I'm more comfortable with animals than with people.
>
> I would love to meet you because I have many questions for you and would love to just talk for a few minutes in person. Is there any way for me to visit with you, even briefly, at your place in Massachusetts?
>
> Please say Hi to your fox, Teacup, for me.
>
> I hope to hear from you.
>
> Best regards,
> Sharon Valero

After some sleuthing, I was able to contact Corwin's publicist who agreed to put the letter in his hands. He responded within a day. Not long after, Jeff Corwin hosted Sharon during a show he put on for a fair in Massachusetts, taking her "backstage" and letting her hold several animals, including Teacup.

The next day, Sharon's mother was breathless over the phone as she told me about the visit. She said I would not have recognized her daughter—not only because she had shampooed, blow-dried, and brushed her hair, and freshly filed and polished her nails, but because she was shy, quiet, polite, and "on her very best behavior!"

When I next saw Sharon—it was just two weeks later that she was again admitted to the hospital—physically she felt lousy, but emotionally she was still glowing from the visit. "It was the best day of my life!" she told me.

Between spasms of coughing, she smiled and showed me pictures her mother had taken of her with Jeff Corwin. I was already beaming when, for the first time I had known her, she opened her arms and gave me a big hug.

Witnessing and sharing in Sharon's joy meant that we were both having a very good day. The process of trying to come up with something that could ease Sharon's distress or meaningfully brighten her gloomy life was not in any algorithm or best-practice guideline. It was rooted in imagining opportunities rather than responding to problems.

The Importance of Centering Practice

Making use of therapeutic imagination depends on our ability to remain fully present. Of course, clinical practice rarely occurs in a meditative milieu. In contemporary palliative-care practice, there are usually one or more consults to be performed, a phone call that needs to be made to the son and daughter-in-law of a patient in the ICU, and a few calls to be returned to colleagues. The assault on the clinician's emotions, schedule, sights, and smells can make maintaining any sense of equilibrium a challenge. Centering practice cultivates a clinician's capacity to bend and absorb, recoil and endure.

To do this work effectively while honoring healthy psychological and ethical boundaries, we must at once be able to imagine the world of the other, while at the same time remaining mindful that our only purpose in the encounter is to serve.

I am at my best as a doctor when I can remain grounded and still—even in the midst of acting swiftly—listening deeply, keeping my heart open, and remembering to breathe.

Acknowledgments

We acknowledge that it took a multitude of support to bring this work to fruition. Blessings to Ira Byock, Doen Daggy, Nick Flynn, Marie Howe, Dawn King, and John Maradik, for their specific, caring help; Rita Sherr and Steve Glass, for being guardians of this work; Joshua Milton Moses, for his friendship and inspiration; and the Garrison Institute for hosting our symposiums and bringing so many wonderful caregivers together. Our fearless editor, Laura Cunningham, and the team at Wisdom Publications, for being wonderful partners; Lorraine Weingast, Joel Weingast, Richard Ellison, and Kenya Paley, for being our parents; Trudi Jinpu Hirsch for her wisdom and guidance, Enkyo O'Hara for her teachings, and Mary Remington and Dr. Martin Ehrlich for their commitment to NYZCCC from the beginning; Rozanne Gold, Richard Stegman, Georgiana Shoren Thomas, Craig Davis, Constance Collins, and Barbara Gallay, for being stewards of the Zen Center mission; Dojun O'Connor, Doji Reigeluth, James Morgan, Melissa Amdur, Evan Zazula, and Doshin Ende, for mentoring others into this path; Dorothy Dai En Friedman, for being a spiritual friend and teacher; and Robert Chodo Campbell, for his authenticity and love.

Thank you to Diane Meier, Bhikkhu Bodhi, Judy Lief, Craig D. Blinderman, Joseph Goldstein, Michael Kearney and Radhule Weininger, Norman Fischer, Joshua Bright, Gil Fronsdal, Kirsten DeLeo, Stephen and Ondrea Levine, Betsey MacGregor, Fernando Kogen Kawai, Robert Chodo Campbell, Shodo Harada, and Ira Byock for the beautiful essays they offered for this book.

Thank you to the Gay Buddhist Fellowship for helping find Issan Dorsey's Dharma Talk. Thank you to all the patients we care for, for your stories, and thank you to all the dedicated staff throughout the world who engage in the work of healing on a daily basis.

Rachel Naomi Remen's stories are from *Kitchen Table Wisdom* by Rachel Naomi Remen, MD, Riverhead Books, 1996; and *My Grandfather's Blessings*, by Rachel Naomi Remen, MD, Riverhead Books, 2001.

right © 1997 by Marie Howe. Used by permission of W. W. Norton & Company, Inc.

"The Layers" copyright © 1978 by Stanley Kunitz, "Passing Through" copyright © 1985 by Stanley Kunitz, "Touch Me" copyright © 1995 by Stanley Kunitz, from *The Collected Poems* by Stanley Kunitz. Used by permission of W. W. Norton & Company, Inc.

Tony Hoagland, "Lucky" and "Medicine" from *Donkey Gospel*. Copyright © 1998 by Tony Hoagland. Reprinted with the permission of The Permissions Company, Inc. on behalf of Graywolf Press, Minneapolis, Minnesota, www.graywolfpress.org.

Naomi Shihab Nye, "Kindness" from *Words Under the Words: Selected Poems*. Copyright © 1995 by Naomi Shihab Nye. Reprinted with the permission of the author.

"Love after Love" from *Collected Poems 1948–1984* by Derek Walcott. Copyright © 1986 by Derek Walcott. Reprinted by permission of Farrar, Straus and Giroux, LLC (rights@fsgbooks.com).

From *Living in the Light of Death: On the Art of Being Truly Alive*, by Larry Rosenberg, pp. 78–122, © 2000 by Larry Rosenberg. Reprinted by arrangement with The Permissions Company, Inc., on behalf of Shambhala Publications, Inc., Boston, MA. www.shambhala.com.

Mark Doty's "The Embrace." From *Sweet Machine*, published by HarperCollins. Copyright © 1998 by Mark Doty. All rights reserved. Used with permission.

"Turtle, Swan," by Mark Doty. Reprinted by permission of David R. Godine, Publisher, Inc. Copyright © 1987 by Mark Doty.

"For the Anniversary of My Death" and "Separation" from *The Second*

Four Books of Poems by W. S. Merwin. Copyright © 1992 by W. S. Merwin, used with permission of The Wylie Agency LLC.

Thank you to Wisdom Publications for permission to use "Creating Our Dharma Vision" by Anyen Rinpoche from *Dying with Confidence*, 2014; "Our Real Home" by Ajahn Chah from *Food for the Heart: The Collected Teachings of Ajahn Chah*, 2002; and "Acknowledging the Shadow" by Rodney Smith from *Lessons from the Dying*, 2015.

Polishing the Mirror: How to Live from Your Spiritual Heart by Ram Dass. Copyright © 2013 by the Love Serve Remember Foundation. Published with permission by Sounds True.

"Unfinished Business, and How You Know That You Know" by Elisabeth Kübler-Ross. Copyright ©1982 by The Elisabeth Kübler-Ross Family LP. Reprinted by arrangement with The Elisabeth Kübler-Ross Family LP and The Barbara Hogenson Agency. All rights reserved. For more information on Dr. Elisabeth Kübler-Ross, please visit: www.ekrfoundation.org.

Bibliography

Aitken, Robert. *Taking the Path of Zen*. New York: North Point Press, 1982.

Beck, Joko. *Nothing Special*. New York: Harper One, 1994.

Buksbazen, John. *Zen Meditation in Plain English*. Boston, MA: Wisdom Publications, 2002.

Byock, Ira. *The Best Care Possible: A Physician's Quest to Transform Care through the End of Life*. New York: Avery, 2012.

———. "Conceptual Models and the Outcomes of Caring." *Journal of Pain and Symptom Management* 17, no. 2 (1999): 83–92.

———. *Dying Well: The Prospect for Growth at the End of Life*. New York: Riverhead Books, 1997.

———. "The Nature of Suffering and the Nature of Opportunity at the End of Life." *Clinics in Geriatric Medicine* 12, no. 2 (1996): 237–52.

———. "When Suffering Persists." *Journal of Palliative Care* 10, no. 2 (1994): 8–13.

Byock, Ira, and Joan M. Teno and Marilyn J. Field. "Measuring Quality of Care at Life's End." *Journal of Pain and Symptom Management* 17 no. 2 (1999): 73–74.

Cassel, Eric J. "The Nature of Suffering and the Goals of Medicine." *New England Journal of Medicine* 306, no. 11 (1982): 639–45.

Charon, Rita. *Narrative Medicine: Honoring the Stories of Illness.* Oxford University Press, 2008.

Chochinov, Harvey Max. "Dignity and the Essence of Medicine: The A, B, C, and D of Dignity Conserving Care." *British Medical Journal* 335, no. 7612 (2007): 184–87.

Chochinov, Harvey Max, and Thomas Hassard, Susan McClement,

et al. "The Patient Dignity Inventory: A Novel Way of Measuring Dignity-Related Distress in Palliative Care." *Journal of Pain and Symptom Management* 36, no. 6 (2008): 559–71.

Chodron, Pema. *When Things Fall Apart: Heart Advice for Difficult Times*. Boston: Shambhala Publications, 1997.

Clark, David. "Total Pain: Disciplinary Power and the Body in the Work of Cicely Saunders, 1958–1967." *Social Science Medicine* 49, no. 6 (1999): 727–36.

Dass, Ram, and Paul Gorman. *How Can I Help? Stories and Reflections on Service*. New York: Knopf Publishing Group, 1985.

De Hennezel, Marie. *Intimate Death: How the Dying Teach Us How to Live*. New York: Vintage, 1998.

Doty, Mark. *Heaven's Coast: A Memoir*. New York: Harper Perennial, 1997.

Fischer, Norman. *Taking our Places: The Buddhist Path to Truly Growing Up*. New York: Harper One, 2004.

Frankl, Viktor. *Man's Search for Meaning*. Boston: Beacon Press, 2006.

Gyalwa Kalzang Gyatso (seventh Dalai Lama). "Meditations on the Ways of Impermanence." In *Living in the Face of Death*, edited by Glenn H. Mullin. Ithaca, NY: Snow Lion Publications, 1998.

Harrington, Anne. *The Cure Within: A History of Mind Body Medicine*. New York: W. W. Norton & Company. 2009.

Kabat-Zinn, Jon. *Wherever You Go, There You Are: Mindfulness Meditation in Everyday Life*. NY: Hyperion Publications, 2005.

Kornfield, Jack. *A Path with Heart*. NY: Bantam, 1993.

Longaker, Christine. *Facing Death and Finding Hope: A Guide to the Emotional and Spiritual Care of the Dying*. New York: Doubleday, 1997.

Maezumi, Taizan. *Appreciate Your Life: Zen Teachings of Taizan Maezumi Roshi*. Boston: Shambhala Publications, 2001.

Mahaparinibbana Sutta, Digha Nikaya 16.

Mount, Bal, and John Scott. "Wither Hospice Evaluation." *Journal of Chronic Disease* 36, no. 11 (1983): 731–36.

Puchalski, Christina. A talk given to the students of Spiritual Care

Program's *Contemplative End-of-Life Care* at George Washington University, Washington DC, 2013.

Schneider, D. *Street Zen: The Life and Work of Issan Dorsey*. New York: Marlowe & Co., 2000.

Silananda, U. *The Four Foundations of Mindfulness.* Boston: Wisdom Publications, 1990.

Sogyal Rinpoche. "The Buddhist Sense of Time for the Year 2000." A talk given at the International Palliative Congress, Montreal, September 14, 1998.

Staton, Jana, and Roger Shuy and Ira Byock. *A Few Months to Live*. Washington, DC: Georgetown University Press, 2001.

Steinhauser, Karen E., and Stewart C. Alexander, Ira R. Byock, Linda K. George, Maren K. Olsen, and James A. Tulsky. "Do Preparation and Life Completion Discussions Improve Functioning and Quality of Life in Seriously Ill Patients? Pilot Randomized Control Trial." *Journal of Palliative Medicine* 11, no. 9 (2008): 1234–40.

———. "Seriously Ill Patients Discussions of Preparation and Life Completion: An Intervention to Assist with Transition at the End of Life." *Palliative and Supportive Care* 7, no. 4 (2009): 393–404.

Index

B

E

G

H

N

S

T

Y

Z

About the Contributors

Anyen Rinpoche was born in Amdo, Tibet. His lineage can be traced back directly to the renowned Dzogchen master Patrul Rinpoche, author of *Words of My Perfect Teacher*. Anyen Rinpoche's training included more than fourteen years of intensive study combined with solitary retreat before he obtained the degree of *khenpo* (master teacher) and became the head scholar of his monastic university in Kham, Tibet. Rinpoche is known for his profound understanding of the scriptures as well as his easy-to-understand interpretation of them. He has taught extensively in Tibet and China and now mentors students throughout Southeast Asia, Japan, and North America. He's the author of *Dying with Confidence*, *Journey to Certainty*, and *Momentary Buddhahood*.

Coleman Barks was born and raised in Chattanooga, Tennessee, and educated at the University of North Carolina and the University of California at Berkeley. He taught poetry and creative writing at the University of Georgia for thirty years. He is the author of numerous Rumi translations and has been a student of Sufism since 1977. His work with Rumi was the subject of an hour-long segment in Bill Moyers's *Language of Life* series on PBS, and he is a featured poet and translator in Bill Moyers's poetry special "Fooling with Words." Coleman Barks is a father of two children and the grandfather of five. He lives in Athens, Georgia.

Craig D. Blinderman, MD, is the director of the Adult Palliative Medicine Service at Columbia University Medical Center and serves on the advisory board for the New York Zen Center for Contemplative

Care. He was previously an attending physician on the Palliative Care Service at the Massachusetts General Hospital and directed the MGH Cancer Pain Clinic. Dr. Blinderman has published articles and chapters on early palliative care in lung cancer patients, medical ethics, existential distress, symptom assessment, and quality of life in chronic lung and heart failure patients, as well as pain management in hematology and oncology patients and patients with a history of substance abuse. He is currently the section editor for Case Discussions in the Journal of Palliative Medicine.

Bhikkhu Bodhi, born Jeffrey Block, is an American Theravada Buddhist monk, ordained in Sri Lanka and currently teaching in the New York/New Jersey area. He was appointed the second president of the Buddhist Publication Society and has translated, edited, and authored several publications, including *In the Buddha's Words: An Anthology of Discourses from the Pali Canon*. Bhikkhu Bodhi is the founder of the Buddhist Global Relief organization, which is fighting hunger across the world.

Joshua Bright is an award-winning photojournalist who works for the *New York Times*, *Vogue* magazine, and many other publications and organizations. Joshua has been a recipient of multiple photography awards including, in 2014, two Best of Photojournalism awards, a Pictures of the Year International Award of Excellence, and inclusion in the *American Photography 30* book. He has taught photography at various levels, most recently at the prestigious Maine Media Workshops and Alfred University.

Ira Byock, MD, is director of Palliative Medicine at Dartmouth-Hitchcock Medical Center and a professor of Anesthesiology and Community and Family Medicine at Dartmouth Medical School. His first book, *Dying Well*, has become a standard in the field of end-of-life care. His most recent book, *The Four Things That Matter Most*, is used as a counseling tool widely by palliative care and hospice programs, as well as within pastoral care. A consistent advocate for the voices and rights of dying patients and their families, Dr. Byock has been the recipient of many awards, including the National Hospice Organization's Person of the Year, and the Outstanding Colleague Award of the National Association of Catholic Chaplains.

Robert Chodo Campbell cofounded the New York Zen Center for Contemplative Care, the first Buddhist organization to offer fully accredited chaplaincy training in America. The organization delivers contemplative approaches to care through education, direct service, and meditation practice. Chodo is part of the core faculty for the Buddhist track in the Master in Pastoral Care and Counseling at the New York Theological Seminary. He is codirector of Contemplative Care Services for the Department of Integrative Medicine at Beth Israel Medical Center. His groundbreaking work has been widely featured in the media, including the PBS Religion and Ethics Newsweekly blog, and in numerous print publications such as the *New York Times* and *Los Angeles Times*. He was also a contributing writer in *The Arts of Contemplative Care: Pioneering Voices in Buddhist Chaplaincy and Pastoral Work*.

Rafael Campo, MD, attended Amherst College and Harvard Medical School before publishing his first collection of poems, *The Other Man Was Me: A Voyage to the New World*, which won the National Poetry Series Open Competition. Since then, he has published several books and has recently received fellowships from the Guggenheim Foundation and the Echoing Green Foundation. He is a practicing physician at Harvard Medical School and the Beth Israel Deaconess Medical Center in Boston.

Ajahn Chah was Thailand's best-known meditation teacher, renowned for the beauty and simplicity of his teachings. His charisma and wisdom influenced many American and European seekers, and helped shape the American Vipassana community. He is the author of *Food for the Heart*.

Ram Dass has made his mark on the world giving teachings and promoting loving service, harmonious business practices, and conscious care for the dying. The author of the seminal 1971 work *Be Here Now*, his influence has extended over four generations of spiritual seekers. He lives in Maui.

Kirsten DeLeo is the International Training Manager and Senior Educator for the Spiritual Care Education Program. Drawing from more than fifteen years of experience accompanying people in the last phase of life, Kirsten leads trainings for professionals and the public, and is faculty for Naropa University's 'Contemplative End of Life Care' training. She is a counselor specializing in spiritual care and in supporting people living with illness. Kirsten completed a three-year meditation retreat under the guidance of Sogyal Rinpoche and is a Senior Meditation Instructor in Rigpa.

Issan Dorsey, born Tommy Dorsey, Jr., was a Soto Zen monk and teacher, Dharma heir of Zentatsu Richard Baker, and onetime abbot of Hartford Street Zen Center (HSZC) located in the Castro district of San Francisco. He died of complications from AIDS in 1990. He established the Maitri Hospice at HSZC for students and friends dying of AIDS during the spread of the epidemic in the 1980s—the first Buddhist hospice of its kind in the United States. The book *Street Zen* is inspired by his life and journey.

Mark Doty is the author of many poetry collections, including *Fire to Fire: New and Selected Poems*, which won the National Book Award for Poetry in 2008. He is also the author of four volumes of nonfiction prose, including a New York Times bestseller. Doty's work has been honored by the National Book Critics Circle Award, the Los Angeles Times Book Prize, a Whiting Writers Award, two Lambda Literary Awards, and the PEN/Martha Albrand Award for First Nonfiction. Doty lives in New York City. He is Professor/Writer in Residence at Rutgers University in New Brunswick, New Jersey.

Norman Fischer is a Zen Buddhist priest and teacher. He earned an MFA from the University of Iowa Writers' Workshop and an MA from the Graduate Theological Union at the University of California, Berkeley. An author of both poetry and nonfiction, Fischer has also written numerous books on spirituality, among them *Opening to You: Zen-Inspired Translations of the Psalms*, *Taking Our Places: The Buddhist Path to Truly Growing Up*, and *Pitfalls*, *Training in Compassion: Zen Teachings on the Practice of Lojong*. Fischer was coabbot for the San Francisco Zen Center from 1995 to 2000. He is a founder of and teacher at the Everyday Zen Foundation.

Nick Flynn is the author of the poetry collections *The Captain Asks for a Show of Hands*, *Blind Huber,* and *Some Ether,* which was the recipient of the PEN/Joyce Osterweil Award. He is also the author of the memoir *Another Bullshit Night in Suck City*, which received the PEN/Martha Albrand Award, has been widely translated, and was adapted into the film *Being Flynn*. He teaches part-time at the University of Houston and lives in Brooklyn, New York.

Gil Fronsdal is a coteacher at the Insight Meditation Center in Redwood City, California. He has practiced Zen and Vipassana in the United States and Asia since 1975. He was a Theravada monk in Burma in 1985 and in 1989 began training with Jack Kornfield to teach Vipassana. In 1998 he received a PhD in religious studies from Stanford University, studying the earliest developments of the bodhisattva ideal. He is the author of *The Issue at Hand*, *A Monastery Within*, and *Unhindered* and is the translator of *The Dhammapada*.

Joseph Goldstein has been leading insight and lovingkindness meditation retreats worldwide since 1974. He is a cofounder of the Insight Meditation Society in Barre, Massachusetts, where he is one of the organization's guiding teachers. He is the author of *Mindfulness: A Practical Guide to Awakening*, *A Heart Full of Peace*, *Insight Meditation: The Practice of Freedom*, and many other titles.

Shodo Harada Roshi is abbot of Sogen-ji, a three-hundred-year-old Rinzai Zen monastery in Okayama, Japan. He is a master of Japanese calligraphy and has conducted demonstrations at the Asian Art Museum in San Francisco and the Metropolitan Museum in New York. He is also abbot of Tahoma Monastery on Whidbey Island north of Seattle. He founded Enso House, a hospice affiliated with Tahoma, where his students attend to the dying.

Tony Hoagland was born in 1953 in Fort Bragg, North Carolina. He earned a BA from the University of Iowa and an MFA from the University of Arizona. Hoagland's books of poetry, including *Sweet Ruin*, *What Narcissism Means to Me*, and *Donkey Gospel*, have won many prizes and accolades. His many honors include fellowships from the National Endowment for the Arts and the Provincetown Fine Arts Work Center, as well as the Poetry Foundation's Mark Twain Award. Hoagland teaches at the University of Houston and in the Warren Wilson MFA program.

Marie Howe was born in Rochester, New York, and attended Sacred Heart Convent School and the University of Windsor before receiving an MFA from Columbia University. Her first collection, *The Good Thief*, was chosen for the National Poetry Series by Margaret Atwood. In 1989, Howe's brother John died of an AIDS-related illness. *What the Living Do*, an elegy to John, was praised by *Publishers Weekly* as one of the five best poetry collections of the year. Howe has taught at Sarah Lawrence College, Columbia, and NYU. She coedited the anthology *In the Company of My Solitude: American Writing from the AIDS Pandemic*.

Fernando Kogen Kawai, MD, is a geriatrician and palliative care physician and works as an attending physician and key faculty member at New York Hospital, Queens. A graduate of the Harvard Geriatrics Fellowship Program at Beth Israel Deaconess Medical Center in Boston, he completed his hospice and palliative medicine fellowship at Stanford University. He presented much of his work at national meetings of the American Geriatrics Society and the American Academy of Hospice and Palliative Medicine. He has been recognized with numerous awards including the New Clinician Educator Award from Harvard Medical School, a Leadership Recognition Award from Stanford University, an award for exceptional humanistic qualities, and a merit of honor for his work with underserved minorities. Fernando lived in Japan and has practiced meditation in Asia and New York.

Michael Kearney, MD, has over thirty years experience in palliative care. He is especially interested in combining medical treatment with approaches that enhance the innate healing capacities of body and mind.

Elisabeth Kübler-Ross, MD, coauthor of *Life Lessons*, earned a place as the best-loved and most respected authority on the subjects of death and dying. Through her many books, as well as her years working with terminally ill children, AIDS patients, and the elderly, Elisabeth Kübler-Ross has brought comfort and understanding to millions coping with their own deaths or the death of a loved one. In 1977 she was chosen as Woman of the Year by *Ladies' Home Journal*. Dr. Kübler-Ross, whose books have been translated into twenty-seven languages, passed away in 2004 at the age of 78. Before Dr. Kübler-Ross's death, she and David Kessler completed work on their second collaboration, *On Grief and Grieving*.

Stanley Kunitz was an award-winning American poet. After studying at Harvard University he worked as an editor and wrote poetry for his first book *Intellectual Things*. After serving in World War II, he began work as a professor and completed his collection *Passports to the War*. He was awarded the Pulitzer Prize in 1959 for his work *Selected Poems 1928–1958*. His later collection *Passing Through* won a National Book Award. He served as Poet Laureate Consultant in Poetry to the Library of Congress from 1974–1976, and again from 2000–2001.

Stephen and Ondrea Levine provided emotional and spiritual support for those who are life-threatened and for caregivers for over thirty-two years. Through their writings, as well as through their healing and forgiveness workshops, Stephen and Ondrea have touched the lives of thousands of people all over the world. They are the authors of numerous books, including *Who Dies*, *Embracing the Beloved*, and *A Year to Live*. Stephen and Ondrea live in northern New Mexico.

Judy Lief is a writer and Buddhist teacher who trained under the Tibetan meditation master Ven. Chögyam Trungpa Rinpoche. She has been a teacher and practitioner for over thirty-five years and continues to teach throughout the world. She is the editor of numerous books on Buddhist meditation and psychology and is the author of *Making Friends with Death: A Buddhist Guide to Encountering Mortality* and numerous articles that have appeared in *The Shambhala Sun*, *Tricycle*, *O Magazine*, *Buddhadharma*, and *The Naropa Journal of Contemplative Psychotherapy*. She offers workshops and retreats on the contemplative care of the dying for pastoral counselors, hospice workers, caregivers, and medical personnel.

Betsy MacGregor, MD, is an advocate of integrative, patient-centered medical care. Having been a cancer patient in her own hospital, she has a deep appreciation for the miraculous gift that life truly is. For nearly thirty years Betsy was a senior staff pediatrician and director of adolescent medicine at Beth Israel Medical Center, a major academic medical center in New York City, where she founded and directed the Pediatric Pain Management Program and the hospital-wide Program for Humanistic and Complementary Health Care. In addition, as a George Soros Faculty Scholar with the Open Society Institute's Project on Death in America, she designed and directed a three-year research project entitled Dying and the Inner Life, aimed at learning from people with terminal illness about what it means to face the reality of one's own dying.

Diane E. Meier, MD, is director of the Center to Advance Palliative Care, a national organization devoted to increasing the number and quality of palliative care programs in the United States. Under her leadership the number of palliative care programs in US hospitals has more than tripled in the last ten years. She is also vice-chair for Public Policy, Professor of Geriatrics and Palliative Medicine, and Gaisman Professor of Medical Ethics at the Icahn School of Medicine at Mount Sinai in New York City. In 2009–2010, she was a Health and Aging Policy Fellow in Washington, DC. Awards include a MacArthur Foundation "genius award" Fellowship in 2008; HealthLeaders recognition as one of twenty Americans who make health care better in 2010; the American Cancer Society's 2012 Medal of Honor for Cancer Control in recognition of her pioneering leadership; and the American Geriatrics Society Edward Henderson State-of-the-Art Lecture Award in 2013.

W. S. Merwin is known for his poetry's distinctive, sparse style, and his condemnation of the Vietnam War and destruction of the environment. Merwin has published more than thirty books of poetry, translation, and prose. He's also garnered two Pulitzer prizes for *The Carrier of Ladders* in 1971 and *The Shadow of Sirius* in 2009.

Naomi Shihab Nye was born in 1952 in St. Louis, Missouri. In her writing, she has been inspired by her experiences as an Arab-American, as well as by richness and diversity of the people and places she has encountered, both in the American Southwest and abroad. She has gone on to write several poetry collections, essays, and novels, including her collection *19 Varieties of Gazelle: Poems of the Middle East*, which was a finalist for the National Book Award. Her many honors include four Pushcart Prizes, a Jane Addams Children's Book Award, a Paterson Poetry Prize, a Guggenheim Fellowship, and a Lannan Fellowship. She lives in San Antonio, Texas.

Frank Ostaseski is a Buddhist teacher, international lecturer, and leading voice in contemplative end-of-life care. In 1987, he cofounded the Zen Hospice Project, the first Buddhist hospice in America. In 2004, he created the Metta Institute to provide innovative educational programs and trainings that foster compassionate, mindfulness-based care. In 2001, Frank was honored by the Dalai Lama for his years of service to the dying and their families. In 2003, he was named one of America's fifty most innovative people in America by the AARP magazine. Frank has served as a consultant to several healthcare organizations, NGOs, and foundations including the Robert Wood Johnson Foundation, the Fetzer Institute, and others. Frank is also the author of the Being a Compassionate Companion audio series.

Rachel Naomi Remen, MD, is clinical professor of Family and Community Medicine at the University of California San Francisco School of Medicine and founder and director of the Institute for the Study of Health and Illness at Commonweal. She is considered one of the pioneers of Integrative Medicine and Relationship Centered Care. Her discovery model curriculum, the Healer's Art, enables medical students to embrace the values of their lineage and is taught at eighty medical schools nationally as well as at schools in seven countries abroad. Dr. Remen's bestselling books, *Kitchen Table Wisdom: Stories that Heal* and *My Grandfather's Blessings: Stories of Strength, Refuge and Belonging*, have been translated into twenty-one languages. Dr. Remen has a sixty-year personal history of Crohn's disease, and brings the perspective and wisdom of both physician and patient to her work.

Larry Rosenberg is an American Buddhist teacher who founded the Cambridge Insight Meditation Center in Cambridge, Massachusetts, where he is also a resident teacher. He is also a senior teacher at the Insight Meditation Society in Barre, Massachusetts. Rosenberg was a professor of psychology at the University of Chicago and Harvard Medical School until, disappointed with his experience with academia, he turned to intensive Buddhist practice. His book *Breath by Breath* is a clear description of the practice of *anapanasati* (mindful breath meditation). His emphasis on the breath as an object of meditation was, in part, inspired by his encounter with the Thai meditation teacher Buddhadasa and informs his teachings in Insight Meditation.

Jalāl ad-Dīn Muhammad Rūmī, more popularly simply Rūmī, was a thirteenth-century Persian poet, jurist, Islamic scholar, theologian, and Sufi mystic who was concerned with the spiritual evolution and consciousness of human beings. He is one of the most widely read poets in the United States and around the world.

Dame Cicely Saunders was a nurse and social worker born in Barnet, England, in 1918. During the late 1940s, she started working with terminally ill patients. She founded the first modern hospice, St. Christopher's Hospice, in 1967 to provide palliative care to those in need, promoting the principle of dying with dignity. In 1979, Queen Elizabeth II honored Cicely Saunders with the title Commander of the Order of the British Empire, and in 1989 was appointed by the Queen to the Order of Merit. For nearly twenty years, she served as the medical director of St. Christopher's Hospice.

Senryu was the first to write haiku in the light style named after him. For decades he was esteemed as the foremost haiku critic in Edo. He would rate every haiku presented to him, and those he judged best were published in a series of pamphlets. It is estimated that he criticized about two and a half million poems in his lifetime. Senryu's name consists of the characters for stream (*sen*) and willow (*ryu*). These signs appear in his death poem with their Japanese pronunciations, *kawa* and *yanagi*.

Jason Shinder is a poet and editor, who grew up in Brooklyn and Merrick, New York. Shinder is the author of three collections of poetry: *Stupid Hope*, *Among Women*, and *Every Room We Ever Slept In*, a New York Public Library Notable Book. Shinder's stark yet lyrical poems are often concerned with loss, joy, and the vulnerable intimacy of relationships. His honors include a fellowship from the National Endowment for the Arts and the post of poet laureate of Provincetown, Massachusetts. He was the founding director of the YMCA's National Writer's Voice—a national network of literary arts centers—and a writing program for the Sundance Institute. He later became the YMCA's director of arts and humanities. He also taught at Bennington College and the New School University. After a battle with lymphoma and leukemia, Shinder died in Manhattan at the age of fifty-two.

Derek Walcott was awarded the Nobel Prize for Literature in 1992, two years after the publication of his most ambitious and celebrated work to date, "Omeros," an epic poem which draws on the Homeric tradition and relocates it in the voices and lives of the people of the Caribbean. With over twenty collections spanning four decades, Walcott is a towering and influential presence in contemporary poetry. He is an honorary member of the American Academy and the Institute of Arts and Letters, and was awarded the Queen's Gold Medal for Poetry in 1988. His collection "White Egrets" won the 2010 T. S. Eliot Prize.

Radhule B. Weininger, MD, works with the spiritually homeless and disappointed, individuals who want to find their own sense of spiritual connectedness. She specializes in seeing clients from international and minority backgrounds, helping them to bridge cultural and religious identities. She has been studying mindfulness meditation, both as a personal practice and as a tool in psychotherapy, for thirty years. Her current teachers are Jack Kornfield and B. Alan Wallace. She is on the faculty of the Anamcara Institute for Spiritual End of Life Care. Her husband, Michael Kearney, MD, a palliative care physician, and she are authors of several book chapters and a JAMA article on whole-person care, spiritual care, and mindfulness meditation. Together they teach at conferences, seminars, and retreats both nationally and internationally.

About the Editors

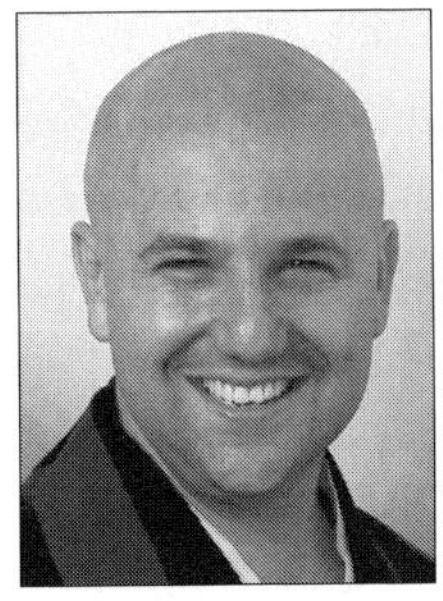

Rev. Dr. Paley Ellison, MFA, LMSW, DMIN, cofounded the New York Zen Center for Contemplative Care, the first Zen-based organization to offer fully accredited ACPE clinical chaplaincy training in America, which delivers contemplative approaches to care through education, direct service, and meditation practice. Paley Ellison is the academic advisor for the Buddhist students in the Master in Pastoral Care and Counseling program at NYZCCC's education partner, New York Theological Seminary. He has served as the codirector of Contemplative Care Services for the Department of Integrative Medicine and as the chaplaincy supervisor for the Pain and Palliative Care Department at Mount Sinai Beth Israel Medical Center, where he also served on the Medical Ethics Committee. He is currently on the faculty of the University of Arizona Medical School's Center for Integrative Medicine's Integrative Medicine Fellowship, and he is a visiting professor at the McGovern Center for Humanities and Ethics, of the University of Texas Health Science Center of Houston Medical School.

Paley Ellison is a dynamic, original, and visionary leader and teacher. His public programs have introduced thousands to the practices of mindful and compassionate care of the living and dying. More than 30,000 people listen to his podcasts each year. He has lectured and held contemplative care trainings and retreats at leading institutions in the fields of medicine and contemplative practice, including Harvard Divinity School, Mount Sinai Medical Center, Union Theological

Seminary, University of Arizona Medical School, Naropa University, Omega Institute, Barre Center for Buddhist Studies, The Rubin Museum of Art, and many others. Koshin is a popular keynote speaker for national conferences, including the National Hospice and Palliative Care Organization, Association of Clinical Pastoral Education, Integrative Healthcare Symposium, and the Palliative Care Symposium.

His groundbreaking work has been widely featured in the media, including the PBS Religion and Ethics Newsweekly, and in numerous print publications such as the *New York Times* and *Los Angeles Times*. He is the coauthor of the chapter "Rituals and Resilience" in the book *Creating Spiritual and Psychological Resilience* (Routledge, 2009). He also authored the chapter "The Jeweled Net: What Dogen and the Avatamsaka Sutra Can Offer Us as Spiritual Caregivers" in the book *The Arts of Contemplative Care: Pioneering Voices in Buddhist Chaplaincy and Pastoral Work* (Wisdom Publications, 2012). He received his clinical training at Mount Sinai Beth Israel Medical Center and the Jungian Psychoanalytic Association. He began is formal Zen training in 1987, and he delightfully continues to study with Dorothy Dai En Friedman, Zen teacher in the White Plum Soto Zen Lineage. He is a senior Zen monk, Zen teacher and student, ACPE supervisor, and Jungian psychotherapist.

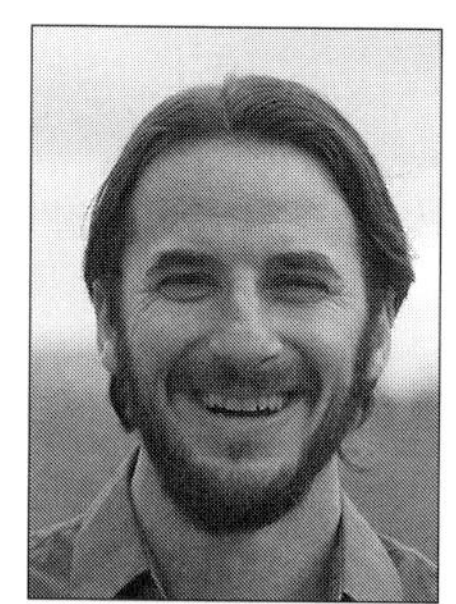

MATT WEINGAST's interest in meditation began when he was in his twenties. In the midst of his travels, he served as a Peace Corps volunteer in Ghana, teaching high school science. Matt received an MFA from the University of Massachusetts–Amherst where he both taught writing and mentored incoming writing instructors. He is currently editor of the Insight Journal and director of communications at Barre Center for Buddhist Studies in Central Massachusetts.

About the New York Zen Center for Contemplative Care

The New York Zen Center for Contemplative Care is the leading organization in both accredited contemplative clinical education and direct care, grounded in Zen practice. NYZCCC is a nonprofit charitable organization dedicated to transforming the way care is offered and received in major medical centers, hospices, and community-based care. We do this work in order to create a more courageous and harmonious world.

To find out more about our programs, visit zencare.org:

- Accredited Clinical Training Programs and Medical Education
- Community Support and Care
- Master in Buddhist Studies Program
- Zen Training

NYZCCC is a 501(c)(3) organization, and all donations in support of our mission are tax deductible.

Also Available from Wisdom Publications

The Arts of Contemplative Care
Pioneering Voices in Buddhist Chaplaincy and Pastoral Work
Edited by Cheryl A. Giles and Willa B. Miller
Foreword by Judith Simmer-Brown
Preface by Pat Enkyo O'Hara

"Courageous contemporary Buddhist practitioners bring the depth of their practice into direct service and healing."—Judith Simmer-Brown, from the foreword

Lessons from the Dying
Rodney Smith
Foreword by Joseph Goldstein

"This is a valuable book of practice, stories, and meditations."—Jack Kornfield, author of *A Path with Heart*

Buddhist Care for the Dying and Bereaved
Edited by Jonathan S. Watts and Yoshiharu Tomatsu

"A valuable and amazing resource! This collection is a 'must' for those of us involved in chaplaincy care."—Pat Enkyo O'Hara, abbot, Village Zendo

How to Enjoy Death
Preparing to Meet Life's Final Challenge without Fear
Lama Zopa Rinpoche

"Knowing how to help others at the time of death is such important education to have. By providing the right support, the right environment, you can help your loved one die peacefully, with virtuous thoughts, and thus have a good rebirth."—Lama Zopa Rinpoche, from the preface

Dying with Confidence
A Tibetan Buddhist Guide to Preparing for Death
Anyen Rinpoche
Translated by Allison Choying Zangmo

"A powerful guidebook and a source of comfort at life's most crucial moment."—Tulku Thondup Rinpoche, author of *Boundless Healing*

Wholesome Fear
Transforming Your Anxiety about Impermanence and Death
Lama Zopa Rinpoche and Kathleen McDonald

"This book is a powerful reminder of the gift of the truth of impermanence. It is a veritable treasure in the literature on being with dying."
—Joan Halifax

How to Live Well with Chronic Pain and Illness
A Mindful Guide
Toni Bernhard

"The overarching message for those with chronic illness—and for all the rest of us as well—is that self-compassion is the most reliable refuge."
—Sylvia Boorstein, author of *Happiness Is an Inside Job*

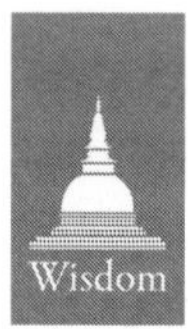

About Wisdom Publications

Wisdom Publications is the leading publisher of classic and contemporary Buddhist books and practical works on mindfulness. To learn more about us or to explore our other books, please visit our website at wisdompubs.org or contact us at the address below.

Wisdom Publications
199 Elm Street
Somerville, MA 02144 USA

We are a 501(c)(3) organization, and donations in support of our mission are tax deductible.

Wisdom Publications is affiliated with the Foundation for the Preservation of the Mahayana Tradition (FPMT).